Safety

Also in the Growing, Growing Strong:
A Whole Health Curriculum for Young Children Series

Body Care

Fitness and Nutrition

Social and Emotional Well-Being

Community and Environment

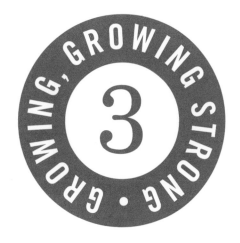

A Whole Health Curriculum for Young Children

Safety

Third Edition

Connie Jo Smith
Charlotte M. Hendricks
Becky S. Bennett

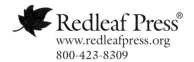

Redleaf Press®
www.redleafpress.org
800-423-8309

Published by Redleaf Press
10 Yorkton Court
St. Paul, MN 55117
www.redleafpress.org

First edition published 1997. Second edition 2006. Third edition 2014.
Cover design by Jim Handrigan
Cover photograph by Blend Images Photography/Veer
Interior design by Percolator
Typeset in Stone Informal, Matrix Script, and Trade Gothic
Illustrations by Chris Wold Dyrud
Printed in the United States of America
20 19 18 17 16 15 14 13   1 2 3 4 5 6 7 8

Library of Congress Cataloging-in-Publication Data
Smith, Connie Jo.
   Safety / Connie Jo Smith, Charlotte M. Hendricks, Becky S. Bennett. — Third edition.
      pages cm — (Growing, growing strong : a whole health curriculum for young children)
   Summary: "The earlier children learn about safety, the more naturally they will develop habits that lead to lifelong patterns of safe behavior. These activities introduce topics such as seat belt use, fire and burn prevention, and tobacco and alcohol awareness in developmentally appropriate ways to help children take care of themselves."— Provided by publisher.
   ISBN 978-1-60554-242-3 (pbk.)
   ISBN 978-1-60554-333-8 (e-book)
   1. Children's accidents—Prevention. 2. Safety education.   I. Hendricks, Charlotte M., 1957- II. Bennett, Becky S., 1954- III. Title.
   HV675.72.S56 2013
   372.37'043—dc23
                                                                                            2013021775

To the memory of my parents, Nevolyn and George. My mother taught me that a sense of humor is an essential life skill, regardless of age. My dad taught me the importance of love and independence.

—Connie Jo

To Gayle Cunningham for guidance and friendship, and to Don Palmer for always being there for me. And in memory of Nic Frising for showing the humor in life through art.

—Charlotte

To the memory of my parents, Charlie and Jeanette, who gave me life, love, and encouragement to follow my dreams. And to my partner, Connie, who has taught me so much about the early care and education field, love, and family.

—Becky

Contents

Acknowledgments

We would like to express heartfelt appreciation to our talented, hardworking, and ever-positive editor, Kyra Ostendorf. This book is much richer for her ideas, guidance, and smiles—those given in person and those that arrived through electronic communication ;-). Thanks to Elena Fultz and Grace Fowler, interns at Redleaf Press, who assisted in technical editing. We are grateful to David Heath for his initial editing support and encouragement. And, of course, we want to acknowledge all the individuals we have had professional encounters with over the years, as each contact has helped us grow and has enhanced our work.

Introduction

Children deserve to live and play in safe environments. Adults have the responsibility to keep children safe; children should not be expected to actively protect themselves. Safety education helps young children develop awareness for a safer life and realize that they can control some aspects of their safety through certain actions. Safety education also helps young children develop skills for safe actions and understand possible consequences of unsafe behavior. The earlier children learn about safety, the more naturally they will develop the attitudes and respect that lead to lifelong patterns of safe behavior.

According to the Centers for Disease Control and Prevention, unintentional injury is the leading cause of death in children (and adults to age forty-four). Because children's cognition is developing, many cannot consistently identify dangerous situations. Also, they often act impulsively, without stopping to consider danger. The goal of safety education, then, is to help children develop safety awareness and learn that they can control some aspects of their safety.

Teach safety in a way that does not frighten children but helps them learn steps to take care of themselves. Help children realize that they can control some aspects of their safety; for example, safe play may prevent injury. Explain that they can make choices to stay safe, just as they wash their hands to prevent disease, and brush their teeth to prevent cavities.

This curriculum will introduce children to lifelong habits that promote safety. Children will gain a higher measure of confidence as they learn about safety and begin to incorporate actions into their lives that make them feel safer. Topics include pedestrian safety, use of seat belts, fire and burn prevention, weapons avoidance, poisoning prevention, and tobacco and alcohol awareness.

Each chapter covers one topic and starts with an overview that includes suggested interest area materials, learning objectives, vocabulary words to introduce and use (which should include vocabulary words in the languages spoken by the families of children in the class), supports for creating the learning environment, and suggestions for evaluating children's understanding of the topic. The overview is followed by activity ideas. Icons appear with each activity to identify the areas of development and learning integrated into the activity:

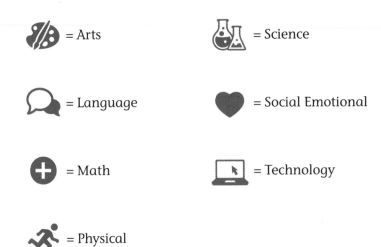

= Arts = Science

= Language = Social Emotional

= Math = Technology

= Physical

Each chapter concludes with a family information page and a take-home family activity page, both of which can be photocopied from the book and distributed to families. These pages can also be downloaded from the Growing, Growing Strong page at www.redleafpress.org for electronic sharing or printing.

INTEREST AREA MATERIALS

Dramatic Play

many kinds of hats and helmets

belts and belt hanger

luggage cart and tie-down

reflective clothing

baby or doll stroller

car safety seats and booster seats

doll high chair with safety strap

flashlights

cellophane paper (red, yellow, green)

empty fire extinguisher without pin

battery-operated candles

rolling pins

bladeless fan

centerpieces

tablecloth

empty, clean rubbing alcohol containers

no-smoking sign

Blocks

many kinds of toy vehicles (fire trucks, buses, trains, airplanes)

toy people to be pedestrians

traffic signs (Stop, Yield, etc.)

road play mat/carpet

string, rope, leather lacing, and yarn

belt buckles for hauling

car garages

small exit signs to use in building

small tornado shelter signs to use in building

Table Toys

transportation puzzles

emergency-related puzzles

building sets with wheels

playhouse vehicles and traffic signs

lacing cards

belts to fasten and unfasten

electric train set

race car set

tabletop road play mat and vehicles

Art

toy vehicles to roll tires through
  painting

green, yellow, and red paint

green, yellow, and red paper

fluorescent tempera paint

tools that require caution (stapler,
  scissors, tools to work with clay)

old belts to cut and glue

string, yarn, and rope pieces

clay and photographs of candleholders

buckles to make paint prints

macramé supplies and pattern for belt
  making

soap bars and plastic knives for carving

craft feathers

Language Arts

car and racing magazines

sample speeding and parking tickets

new-car brochures

street maps

directions with pictures for car
  safety seats

belt catalog

emergency supplies catalog

smoke detector in box with directions

fire exit route maps

photographs of fires, tornadoes,
  hurricanes, and volcanoes

photographs of guns and knives

photographs of chefs using knives

photographs of hunters using guns

toxic and poison warning signs

pictures or photographs of smoke-filled
  rooms

Library

Make Way for Ducklings
  by Robert McCloskey

Do Kangaroos Wear Seat Belts?
  by Jane Kurtz

"Fire! Fire!" Said Mrs. McGuire
  by Bill Martin Jr.

*There Was an Old Lady Who Swallowed
  a Fly* by Simms Taback

That's Dangerous! by Francesco Pittau
  and Bernadette Gervais

Impatient Pamela Calls 9-1-1
  by Mary Koski

Science/Math

reflectors to examine and sort

clips, hooks, and other fasteners

toy tires to sort

spools and dowel rods to create axles

toy cars to take apart

smoke detector to take apart

thermometers (without mercury) to examine and compare

visiting classroom pet to feed

tobacco leaves (whole and crumbled) to examine and smell

tobacco leaf in different stages of growth

pet food containers and pet food to count pieces, weigh, and sort

❶ Safety Note: Children should wash hands after handling pet food.

Outdoors

handheld stop signs

reflective vests

playground streets/roads or trike paths to practice crossing

helmets

ropes to create crosswalks

traffic signs (Stop, Yield, One Way)

horns and bells for riding vehicles

flags for riding vehicles

reflectors for riding vehicles

air pump and tires to fill

paper and pencil to issue speeding tickets

pinwheels, weather vane, windmill

fire escape ladder

outdoor thermometer

parachute

drums

tobacco plant

Technology

weather forecast video or multi-touch mobile device application

weather radio

clocks with alarms to set

bladeless fan

recorded sounds of emergency alarms

Sand, Water, and Construction

wooden squares to paint for traffic signs

charred wood

water hose connected to water supply and designated area for using

watering cans to create floods in containers with dirt or sand

waterwheel for water play

water pump for water play

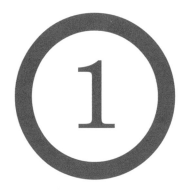

I Want to Be Street-Smart and Street-Safe!

LEARNING OBJECTIVES

- Children will identify traffic personnel.
- Children will demonstrate "stop, look, listen" before crossing the street.
- Children will state that traffic signs and signals are for safety.

Most young children are around moving vehicles on roads and streets to some extent every day of their lives. They may walk to and from school, wait for their bus at the street corner, and run to a neighbor's house down the street to play.

Consider your community and environment when teaching traffic safety. In urban areas, visiting a community park may require crossing a street. Children may play in parking lots or near high-traffic areas that may or may not have pedestrian crossings and traffic signals. In small communities and residential neighborhoods, children often play on sidewalks or driveways and often cross streets to play with neighboring children. Children playing in their own yard or that of a neighbor are probably near a street, and their own driveways have the potential for vehicular traffic.

In rural areas, the greatest danger may be home driveways or dirt roads, or crossing a road to the mailbox. Children must learn to watch not only for cars and trucks but also tractors and other farm equipment.

Several factors put young children at risk for injury as pedestrians. First, a driver may not see a small child who is playing in the street, on a tricycle, or between parked cars. Parents and other family members may be unaware that a child is playing in the driveway, resulting in risk of back-over injury. With large vehicles, such as SUVs and vans, the driver may be unable to see a child playing in front of the vehicle.

To a very young child (under five years of age), the headlights on a vehicle appear to be similar to eyes. They may believe that since they can see the vehicle, the vehicle can see them. Additionally children are impulsive in their actions. If a ball rolls into the street, children are very likely to run after it, possibly in front of a moving vehicle.

Children's sensory development affects their safety. The maturity level of children under ten years of age makes them less able to correctly estimate road dangers or consequences of their actions. For example, preschool children cannot accurately determine if a vehicle is coming toward or going away from them, the distance of the vehicle, or the speed. Family members and other adults often overestimate children's pedestrian skills. A young child can say the words and may appear to "stop, look, and listen" when an adult is supervising. However, young children may misjudge a vehicle's speed or direction and cross in front of an oncoming vehicle.

Adult supervision is essential to child pedestrian safety. Be aware of the potential risks when children are on field trips, entering or exiting a bus or other vehicle, on walks near a street, or on unfenced playgrounds.

VOCABULARY

caution	highway	reflector	traffic
crossing guard	horn	road	vehicle
crosswalk	listen	sidewalk	yellow
driveway	look	sign	yield
flag	parking lot	signal	
green	pedestrian	stop	
helmet	red	street	

CREATING THE ENVIRONMENT

- Create indoor and outdoor play areas to simulate traffic and pedestrian areas. Designate "streets and roads" on the playground pathways so children can practice both pedestrian and vehicle safety awareness.

- Bring in props, such as traffic signs and crossing guard vests, to represent those used in your community.

- Set up a learning center in a large area to represent a street or road crossing, or create a table game with streets, toy vehicles, and figures of people. As children play, encourage them to talk about or clearly show what they are doing ("stop, look, and listen").

■ For child safety, have helmets available for children using riding toys.

■ Prevent children's access to vehicular traffic by using a fenced playground. In high traffic areas or near intersections, provide additional protection against vehicles entering the play area by erecting a concrete barrier or guard rails when possible.

EVALUATION

■ During play, do children pretend to be traffic safety helpers?

■ Are children demonstrating increased awareness of traffic and safety?

■ Are children talking about traffic safety?

■ During play with riding toys, do children increasingly practice traffic rules (for example, stopping at stop signs)?

■ During supervised walks or field trips, do children listen and follow adult instructions regarding traffic safety?

CHILDREN'S ACTIVITIES

Crossing Guards at Work

Use a commercial road play mat/carpet or help children create one. Provide a toy vehicle for each child to place in the road on the mat. Talk about how the vehicles (cars, trucks, buses, and so on) are called traffic, and count the vehicles together. Show the children toy people, and let them know that people are called pedestrians when they are walking along the road. Ask where the pedestrians should stand on the mat. Reinforce that the pedestrians should stand on the sidewalk near crosswalks. Describe a crosswalk and its purpose. Then add a crossing guard to the mat and explain that the crossing guard will help stop the traffic so the pedestrians can cross the street safely. Show children things a crossing guard or traffic police officer might use, like a handheld stop sign or whistle, and items they may wear, such as a safety vest. Let children try on the vest and hold the stop sign.

MATERIALS
- a commercial or classroom-made road play mat/carpet, toy vehicles, toy people, a toy person to represent a crossing guard, a handheld stop sign, a whistle, and a vest or uniform

OTHER IDEAS
- Arrange for children to watch a crossing guard or traffic police officer at work. Take pictures of the event so children can recall more details to use in follow-up activities or role play. Alternatively, watch a short video of a traffic guard at work.

- Invite a crossing guard or traffic police officer to visit the class and demonstrate his work on the trike path, show children his equipment, and answer questions.

- Read and discuss *Make Way for Ducklings* by Robert McCloskey.

- Play and sing the song "She's a Yellow Reflector" by Justin Roberts.

Stop, Look, and Listen

Work with children to create a child-size street scene using cardboard boxes for buildings. Use the trike path, paint, tape, or rope to designate roads with crosswalks. Create sidewalks with flat cardboard or rope. Show children where to stand on the sidewalk, with their toes completely on the sidewalk and not hovering over the curb. Demonstrate how they should look left, look right, and then look left again while listening for any traffic. Show them how they should walk swiftly, but not run, straight across the street to the other side. After children have practiced with you several times, designate half of the children as cars and encourage them to walk the "road" making car sounds. Let the other half of the children practice being safe pedestrians by crossing the street safely. Reverse roles so all children have a turn at practicing pedestrian safety. Remind children that they should only cross real roads if they are with an adult or if their parents or guardians say they can cross without them.

MATERIALS
- cardboard boxes, paint, rope, and tape

OTHER IDEAS

- Sing with children safety songs like "Stop, Look, and Listen/I'm No Fool" by Cliff Edwards.

- Talk about listening for cars and read *Polar Bear, Polar Bear, What Do You Hear?* by Bill Martin Jr.

- Play the traditional children's game Red Light Green Light, a game in which children run when "green light" is called and freeze when "red light" is called. Vary the game by adding walking, jumping, or other movements rather than running. Playing this game without anyone ever being "out" increases the activity time for all and contributes to fitness.

- Play Simon Says, and incorporate commands to stop, look, listen, and go. Increase the difficulty by adding look left, look right, look left again, look behind, go to the crosswalk (on the trike path), and other traffic safety–related actions.

The Driver's View

Tell children that you want them to participate in an experiment, and explain that an experiment is when you try something out to see how it works. Divide the group in half, and let one half of the children walk on the trike path or other designated place while pretending to drive cars, trucks, or buses. Let the other children stand on the shoulder just off of the path or designated "street," and give them balls of different sizes to roll across the "street" while children are "driving" by. Let children exchange roles after a short time. Call everyone together to talk about the experience. Ask what happened. Find out if some balls were harder to see than others when children were driving, and see if they know why. Establish whether it was hard for some drivers to stop and miss the balls. (Were they speeding?) Stress that it is hard for cars to stop quickly, and it is difficult for them to see toys, children, and even short adults. Tell them they should not run into the street for a toy or pet and that it is better to stand and play far away from the street. Explain that they should never play near a car, even a parked car, since a driver who gets in may not see them.

MATERIALS
- medium and large balls

OTHER IDEAS

- Let children ride tricycles instead of walking for the experiment.

- Let children take turns sitting in a parked car with an adult, while another adult places toys in front of or behind the car. Encourage the children inside the car to describe all they can see. Then let the children get out of the car and see the toys that were placed in front or back of the car. Point out that they should not go near cars without an adult or unless their parents or guardians tell them it is all right.

- Read and discuss *The Wheels on the Bus* by Maryann Kovalski.

- Play the traditional children's game Button, Button, Who's Got the Button? to show children that sometimes it is hard to see everything. Relate this to drivers having difficulty seeing children.

Trucking Trike

Display several tricycles or other riding toys for children to examine. Encourage them to look under the trikes and look from all sides. Have children compare and describe the different trikes aloud. Write on a chart what they report. Review with them the names of all the parts (handlebars, seat, pedals, tires, wheels, axle, fender, and others). Show reflectors, and ask what they know about them. Provide several bicycle horns, and let children honk them before asking why people use horns. Wave a bicycle flag, and ask why it is important. Explain how reflectors, horns, and flags are related to safety and may help everyone see and hear tricycles better. Point out that if children see and hear tricycles, it may stop them from running in front of one. Also tell them that these items may help bigger bikes or cars see and avoid hitting trikes.

MATERIALS

- several kinds of tricycles or other riding toys, chart paper, a marker, a variety of reflectors, flags, and various styles of horns

OTHER IDEAS

- Help children attach reflectors, horns, and flags to the classroom tricycles, and during the process discuss the importance of tricycles being seen and heard.

- Provide a photographic display of a variety of bicycles, including a mountain bicycle, racing bicycle, stationary bicycle, tandem bicycle, rickshaw, adult tricycle, recumbent tricycle, and unicycle. Encourage children to examine the photos and discuss safety issues for each. Even better, provide real examples of various bikes for children to examine, and discuss safety issues.

- Visit places that fix or sell bicycles and bicycle accessories, such as tires, wheels, air pumps, reflectors, and horns. Ask the sales clerk to show the children safety-related products.

- Read and discuss *D.W. Rides Again!* by Marc Brown. Listen to "Taking Off My Training Wheels" by Justin Roberts.

Helmets and Hats

Show children a variety of head gear, including hats, caps, and helmets. Ask the children to examine the head gear and talk about what they see. Ask the children which of the items would protect their head best if they had a bike wreck. Talk about the importance of wearing a helmet when riding on a trike, bike, skateboard, scooter, or other riding toy. To follow up, work with each child individually to teach how to put on a helmet properly; then add helmets to the tricycle area for ongoing use.

MATERIALS

- a variety of headgear (including baseball caps, shower caps, straw hats, berets, visors, rain hats, beanies, earmuffs, stocking caps, dress hats, western hats, chief's hats, football helmets, bike helmets, and other head safety gear)

OTHER IDEAS

- Provide old sports magazines so children can look for photographs of protective head gear to use in art projects, such as making a mobile.

- Invite an avid bike rider to show children her bike and accessories, including the helmet, and discuss the safety precautions she takes when riding.

- Encourage children to use art supplies to make helmets for the dolls in the classroom. Help them measure and plan their creations. Supply the art interest area with lids of various sizes, tape, string, papier mâché, and other materials suitable for making helmets.

- Take a picture of each child wearing a helmet, and let children use their photo as the cover for a book they make about being a safe trike rider.

Signs, Signs

Display selected international traffic signs. Ask children to tell you what they think each of the signs means and how the sign can help keep people safe. Review with children what each sign means and what *international* means. Give each child a miniature sign and have him find a large matching one from the display.

MATERIALS

- enlarged and laminated pictures of international traffic signs or commercial tricycle path traffic signs (such as Stop, Yield, One Way, No Right Turn, No Left Turn, No U Turn, No Pedestrians, No Bicycles, Traffic Signal Ahead, School Zone, School Xing, Winding Road, Slippery When Wet, Pedestrian Crossing, and Playground) and teacher-made or commercial miniature traffic signs for the block interest area

OTHER IDEAS

- Provide materials and guidance for children to create traffic signs to be used on the playground or in the block interest area, or to be cut into puzzles.

- Place commercial or classroom-made traffic signs on the playground for children to practice following as pedestrians and drivers of riding toys.

- Visit the city or county traffic sign storage facility, and discuss any recognizable signs.

- Take a walk to see, discuss, and practice following traffic signs.

FAMILY INFORMATION

I WANT TO BE STREET-SMART AND STREET-SAFE!

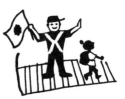

Children are around moving vehicles on roads and streets to some extent every day of their lives. They may walk to and from school, wait for their bus at the street corner, and run to a neighbor's house to play. In rural areas children must learn to watch for not only cars and trucks but also tractors and other farm equipment.

Most young children cannot estimate road dangers or the consequences of their actions. Children under age six do not have the sensory development to judge whether a vehicle is coming toward or going away from them, the distance to the vehicle, or its speed. A child can say and may appear to "stop, look, and listen" when an adult is supervising but may nevertheless cross in front of an oncoming vehicle. To young children, the headlights on a vehicle appear to be similar to eyes. They may believe that if they can see the vehicle, then the driver of the vehicle can "see" them, yet this is not always true.

Supervise your child closely whenever he or she is playing near roads or streets, waiting for a bus, or crossing a street. Check all around your own vehicle before moving from your driveway.

SAFE PLAY AREAS

When your child is playing, she or he may not pay attention to what else is happening. If the ball rolls into the street, your child may run after it. If your child is drawing with chalk in a driveway or alley, he or she probably will not hear or see a car pulling in or out. A child learning to ride a bicycle may turn in front of a moving vehicle.

Look around your home to find the safest areas for your child to play. Your own backyard or driveway, or the sidewalk or cul-de-sac of a quiet neighborhood may prove to be the safest. Some communities have parks and other play areas. Porches and rooftops may also be play areas.

Wherever your child plays, she or he should have adult supervision. Even better, play with your child!

FAMILY ACTIVITY

Find the six people in this picture. What are they doing? Find the five vehicles in the picture. Discuss what happens when people and moving vehicles share the street/road, and what each of the vehicles in this picture will need to do for the safety of everyone.

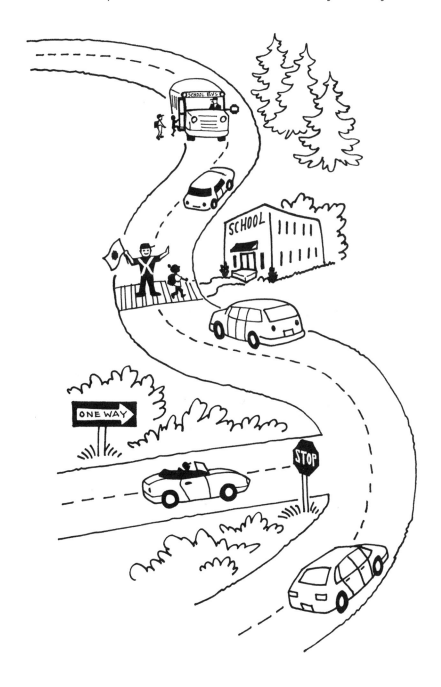

Buckle Me Up!

LEARNING OBJECTIVES

- Children will communicate how seat belts help keep us safe.
- Children will be able to buckle and unbuckle seat belts.
- Children will state that it is a safety rule to buckle up during travel (bus, car).

It's a fact. Seat belts help save lives. According to Safe Kids Worldwide, road injuries are the leading cause of preventable deaths and injuries to children in the United States. Correctly used child safety seats (for example, car seats and booster seats) can reduce the risk of death by up to 71 percent. And it is the law. Child safety seats are required in all fifty states, the District of Columbia, Guam, the Northern Mariana Islands, and the Virgin Islands. Nearly all states require booster seats or other appropriate devices for children who have outgrown their child safety seats but are still too small to use adult seat belts safely. Many other countries, including Australia, Canada, and European countries, have similar requirements.

Remind parents to make sure children are buckled up every time they are in a moving vehicle. Modeling is essential—adults should always buckle up as well!

Teach children that buckling up can help keep them safe. Although children may not understand how staying in the seat protects them, they may understand the consequences of *not* staying in their seat (for example, hitting the dashboard, hitting the windshield, or falling out of the car). Help children begin to understand these consequences, and practice correct use of various child restraints during classroom learning activities and pretend play as well as during transportation.

Remember, too, that in all vehicles, the safest place for infants and children to ride is in the backseat, since that places them farther away from head-on crashes, during which most serious injuries are incurred. Also, most vehicles have air bags in the front seats. These bags inflate at speeds of up to two hundred miles per hour; the impact of an air bag can seriously injure a child, even one buckled in a seat restraint.

Buckle Up Correctly

Child passenger restraint requirements vary from car seat to car seat based on children's age, weight, and height. In all cases, infants use rear-facing infant seats, toddlers use forward-facing child safety seats, and older children use booster seats until they are ready for a seat belt without a booster seat.

Safety seats must be installed correctly in vehicles, and children must be buckled securely. Check with your local police department, health department, or children's hospital to learn more about properly installing child safety seats. Safe Kids Worldwide (www.safekids.org) is a good source of information and safety tips for families and teachers.

Here are some tips for proper safety seat use:

- Choose a safety seat that is right for the child's weight and height. Be sure the seat can be adjusted as the child grows, or purchase a larger seat when needed. When the child outgrows the safety seat, select a booster seat that positions the seat belt and shoulder harness to fit properly over the child's body.

- Remember that every vehicle is different; select a safety seat that can be properly installed in the specific vehicle. Use the car's safety belt or LATCH (Lower Anchors and Tethers for Children) attachment system to lock the safety seat into the car. When properly installed, the safety seat should not move more than one inch side to side or front to back.

- Restrain all children in safety seats when they are in a car with the motor running. Doing so limits their access to power windows, which can cause strangulation injury or death.

- Remember: buckle up properly every time!

VOCABULARY

airplane	click	safety seat	truck
backseat	crash	seat belt	weight
belt	dashboard	snug	windshield
booster seat	detective	strap	wreck
buckle	fasten	tight	
bus	height	train	
car	restraint	tricycle	

CREATING THE ENVIRONMENT

- Provide belts of all kinds for children to practice buckling and unbuckling. If possible, provide seat belts of the type found in most vehicles.

- Transport children only in vehicles that have properly installed safety seats for every child.

- Point out other equipment that has seat belts and safety seats to prevent injury. Strollers, high chairs, grocery store carts, child seats and carriers, and playground seats for very young children are all examples.

- Post a "Buckle Up!" poster. One can be found at www.childhealthonline.org /downloadform.html.

EVALUATION

- Do children discuss the use of seat belts?

- During guided activities, can children buckle and unbuckle seat belts?

- During role-playing, do children practice wearing their seat belts?

- Can children communicate a safety rule for travel in a vehicle (for example, wear a seat belt)?

- When getting into a vehicle, do children initiate buckling up or ask to be buckled up?

CHILDREN'S ACTIVITIES

Belts Galore

Gather a wide variety of belts. Put belts in a large basket, and invite children to examine them. Encourage children to describe and compare the belts. Have them sort the belts many ways (such as by length, width, material, color, and buckle type). Let children try the belts on and practice buckling them. Ask why people wear belts. See if they can think of other kinds of belts. If they do not mention seat belts, point out that people wear seat belts in cars, and ask if they know why. If children mention safety, reinforce this answer. Place some belts in the dramatic play interest area for their role playing and to help them practice with various buckles.

❗ Safety Note: Proceed with caution when using belts, since some families may use a belt to discipline children and thus belts may be frightening. Help children become familiar with the many uses of belts, such as keeping one safe in a car or on a riding toy, holding up one's clothes, and accessorizing clothing.

MATERIALS

■ belts with different kinds of buckles (brass, silver, square, round, or cloth-covered), belts of many colors (brown, tan, black, green, white, multicolored, red, clear), belts made with a variety of materials (braided rope, leather, suede, bead, chain, terry cloth, elastic, silk), belts with accessories (bells, tassels, sequins), and belts that are different widths and lengths

OTHER IDEAS

■ Let children make belts for themselves, dolls, or toy people in the classroom. Provide materials such as fabric and rope, plus buckles for children to attach.

■ Visit a belt factory, leathersmith, or seamstress to see belts being made, and discuss the tools and techniques used.

■ Invite a martial arts instructor to show children the different belts that can be earned, and share information about how meaningful it is to earn each one.

■ Make a classroom chart with each child's name down the left side and family member names across the top (mom, dad, brother, sister, uncle, grandmother, and so on). Ask children to tell you who they know who wears a belt, and help them place an *X* in the appropriate square. Count all *X*s in each column.

Belt Detective

Place several objects that have belts throughout the classroom. Show children one object with a belt, and ask them why they think it has a belt. See if they can think of other objects that might have belts. Encourage them to be a belt detective and search for other types of belts in the room. Let them bring all belted objects together and examine each and discuss the purpose of the belts. When you go on the playground, remind children to be belt detectives and let you know of any belts they find. At the end of the day, encourage children to look for belts at home and every place they go. The next day, ask the children to report on all of the belts they found and what the belts were holding together or keeping safe. If no child mentions seat belts, ask if they saw any.

MATERIALS

- belted objects (such as a stroller, suitcase, backpack, high chair, child car safety seat, child carrier, playground swings, vacuum cleaner belt, lawn mower belt, and car belts)

OTHER IDEAS

- Read and discuss *Monkey with a Tool Belt and the Noisy Problem* by Chris Monroe.

- Let children use a luggage cart and tie-downs to transport boxes.

- Visit a store to look for belted items on display, and discuss the purpose of each.

- Show children where belts are located in a vacuum cleaner, lawn mower, car, or other equipment, and discuss briefly why a belt is needed.

Strolling Sammy

Introduce Sammy, a doll or toy animal, to the children and explain that he wants to go for a ride in the stroller, but he does not want to wear his seat belt. Help the children form two lines facing each other, leaving enough room down the middle for someone to run with the stroller. Select one child to run, pushing the stroller with Sammy, and to stop when she hears a whistle. Blow the whistle to let her know what it sounds like. Have the child who is running begin far enough back from the lined-up children so that she can be running fast before she stops and the children can observe what happens to Sammy. Encourage children to describe any movement Sammy experienced upon stopping. Repeat the activity, giving more children the opportunity to be the runner. Finish the activity by having a child run with Sammy safely buckled in so children can see and discuss the difference. Make the stroller, Sammy, and a space available for all children to experiment during future outdoor times.

MATERIALS

■ a stroller, a doll or stuffed animal, and a whistle

OTHER IDEAS

■ Add Strolling Sofia, a doll securely buckled up, to the Strolling Sammy activity. Let two children run at the same time, one with Sammy and one with Sofia, and compare the different results.

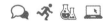

■ Let children sit and lean forward as far as they can toward the floor. Using a measuring tape, measure how far each child can lean without a seat belt. Have children buckle up in a child car safety seat, booster seat, or seat belt, and then measure how far they can lean. Talk about safety implications and how the straps should be snug and untwisted.

■ Provide dolls and stuffed animals for children to take for rides on wheeled toys, and make available belts to secure them.

■ Read and discuss *Do Kangaroos Wear Seat Belts?* by Jane Kurtz.

Click It

Show children a vehicle seat belt, and ask them to tell you what they know about it. Let children examine the belt and practice buckling and unbuckling it. Show the children a car seat and a booster seat, and ask the children what they know about them. Let the children examine them and practice buckling and unbuckling the child car safety seat straps. Tell children that the seat belt and straps should be snug, and let them practice buckling a doll or toy animal in snugly and loosely to see the difference. Stress how important it is for children to sit in a child car safety seat or booster with seat belts in the backseat. Point out that everyone should have their own seat belt, child car safety seat, or booster seat and that no one should share. Allow time for them to practice with more seat belts later.

MATERIALS

- vehicle seat belts (obtained from the police department, a traffic safety school, an automobile salvage lot, or a car garage), a large doll or toy animal, a child car safety seat, and a booster seat

OTHER IDEAS

- Add child car safety seats and dolls, puppets, and toy animals to the dramatic play interest area.

- Assist children in creating a cardboard box vehicle that has seat belts. Use realistic seat belts or child car safety seat straps.

- Visit an airport to see seat belts in planes, hear the preflight information video about seat belts, and practice buckling and unbuckling.

- Play "Come Take a Trip in My Airship" by Natalie Merchant and "Backyard Spaceship" by Justin Roberts, and after moving to the music, ask children if they think spaceships have seat belts.

Seat Belt Marathon

Arrange a trip to a car dealership, and let children examine seat belts, child car safety seats, shoulder straps, and air bag spaces in a variety of vehicles. While at the car dealership, have children practice buckling and unbuckling seat belts in front seats and backseats. Let them know that when a vehicle is moving, they should be in the backseat because it is safer. Assist children in pulling the belts snuggly, and remind them how important that is. Do not allow children to share seat belts, and reinforce that sharing belts is not safe. Help children learn to move the front seat away from the dashboard, and tell them that the farther they are from the dashboard and windshield, the safer they are. Arrange for seats to be removed for children to examine where seat belts are attached. Take photographs of the activities at the dealership so children can reflect on their experience. Help children write and illustrate a thank-you note to the dealership after the trip. Ask whether the dealer would like you to invite the media to the "Seat Belt Marathon." The coverage would be a great thank-you to the dealer and could serve as an excellent public service announcement about the importance of buckling up.

MATERIALS
- a camera, construction paper, paint, and markers

OTHER IDEAS

- As an alternative to the car dealership field trip, ask program employees and families to allow their vehicles to be used for a seat belt marathon on the program premises.

- Print photos from the seat belt marathon activity, and use them for a bulletin board display, in a class book, in children's art projects, and as a handout to send home.

- Play and sing "Yellow Bus" by Justin Roberts. Visit a bus station or a school district transportation department to see if the buses have seat belts, and if they do, practice using them.

- Visit a train station or subway to learn about the seating and safety.

Big Book of Rules to Ride By

Show the children a big blank book, and explain that together you will be creating a book about riding safely in vehicles (cars, trucks, buses, and so on). Write the title on the cover page, "Big Book of Rules to Ride By," and then add your class name as the author and illustrator. Use the date of the activity for the copyright, and explain briefly that this is the date the book was made. Ask children what rules they believe should be in the book, and make the list on chart paper to collect all ideas before you write them in the book. Accept suggestions that children make beyond seat belt safety, since each family may have different rules, such as keeping arms inside the window, no kicking the back of seats, or no screaming. If children do not mention rules you want to include, prompt them with questions or add them as your ideas. Be sure to include the following: use seat belts or car safety seat straps; ride in a car safety seat or booster seat, keeping seat belts or straps snug; ride in the backseat; and make sure all riders have their own seat belts or car safety seat straps. Using the list of ideas, refine and write them in the class book. Designate which children will illustrate the front cover, each page, and the back cover. Take pictures of the children working on the book and also of each book page for an electronic copy of the book that can be printed for each family. Place the finished "Big Book of Rules to Ride By" in the classroom for children to review.

MATERIALS

- several large blank sheets of paper or poster board bound into a book, markers, other art supplies for illustrating, and chart paper

OTHER IDEAS

- Invite a guest from the public transportation or school district transportation department to visit and tell children about bus safety rules. Allow children to role-play—or practice, if a bus is available—getting on a bus and to demonstrate the safety rules.

- Obtain a variety of child car safety seats and booster seats, and check the manufacturer's weight and height requirements of each seat. Weigh and measure each child, and let them know which seats should fit them best. Let children try out the different seats and see how they work and which are comfortable.

- Play and dance to "In the Car" by Justin Roberts and "Bumping Up and Down" by Raffi.

- Engage children in creating a video book about riding safely in vehicles. Take and use photographs of the children, or utilize existing photos in iMovie, Movie Maker, or similar applications.

FAMILY INFORMATION

BUCKLE ME UP!

It's a fact. Seat belts help save lives. Road injuries are the leading cause of preventable deaths and injuries to children in the United States. A collision at only five miles per hour can send an unbuckled child crashing into the dashboard or windshield. According to Safe Kids Worldwide, correctly used child safety seats and booster seats can reduce the risk of death by as much as 71 percent.

Protect your child by putting him or her in the right seat at the right time, and use it according to the manufacturer's directions. Choose one that fits your child based on age, weight, and height. Infants use rear-facing infant seats. Toddlers and young children use forward-facing child safety seats. Older children can use booster seats.

Be sure the car seat can be (or is) properly installed in your vehicle. When properly installed, the car seat should not move more than one inch side to side or front to back. Local Safe Kids coalitions host car seat inspections across the county. Visit www.safekids.org to find an event or assistance in your community.

Make sure your child is correctly buckled up every time she or he is in a vehicle.

THE BACK SEAT IS SAFEST

The safest place for all children to ride is in the backseat. Head-on crashes cause the greatest number of serious injuries. Children riding in the backseat are farthest away from the impact and less likely to be injured or killed. Also, most vehicles now have air bags in the front seats. Air bags inflate at speeds of up to two hundred miles per hour. The impact of an air bag can seriously injure a child in the front seat even if the child is buckled in a car seat or booster seat.

Remember, your child is more likely to buckle up if he or she sees you buckle up.

FAMILY ACTIVITY

Attach this sheet to an empty cereal box, making sure the glue/tape on each square is sufficient for allowing each one to be cut individually. Cut along the dotted lines to make game pieces. To start the matching/memory game, turn the game pieces upside down and distribute them randomly across a flat surface. Assist your child as needed in choosing any two pictures and turning them right side up to see if they match. If there is no match, flip the cards back over, and allow your child to try again. As matches are made, remove those cards. You may also choose to allow the "seat belt" picture to be a "wild card" match to any other card turned over. As the game is played, discuss the importance of "buckling up" to remain safe.

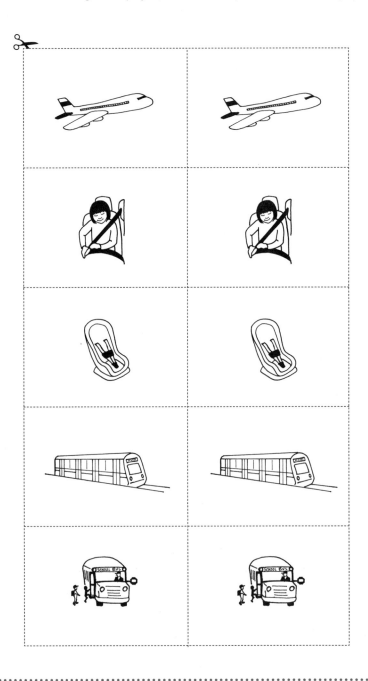

③

My Rules for Emergencies!

LEARNING OBJECTIVES

- Children will practice what to do if they hear a warning alarm (for example, for smoke or a tornado).
- Children will identify and follow exit routes out of their classroom or home.
- Children will describe a type of emergency.

Many types of emergencies can occur at home, in school, or in other environments. Most teachers practice fire evacuation drills, and many teachers prepare for tornadoes, wind events, and earthquakes. A power outage can create an emergency situation and be frightening to children. An alarm or announcement also may warn of a potentially violent situation (for example, lockdown). Know the potential for risk in your area, and help children be prepared.

Young children may be frightened and overwhelmed by discussion of multiple types of emergencies. Begin with basic information—what is an emergency? It is a situation in which you must act quickly or you need immediate help. Build on this information using a single type of emergency, such as fire in the home, school, or some other building.

Young children often die in fires because they do not know what to do. Also, they do not understand that smoke can be as deadly as fire. Teach children to "get low and get out!"

Use appropriate teaching tools for examples and when demonstrating what to do. Children may not understand that fire can go anywhere, and they may try to hide from it. Children may be afraid of firefighters because of their protective clothing and gear. Invite firefighters to visit your classroom in their regular uniforms. Then ask the firefighters to show their gear and put it on while the children are watching. This helps children understand that there is a real person under the mask and helmet. It also reinforces the concept of using safety gear. Likewise, a picture of a person with her clothing on fire may be disturbing to some children. Instead, show a picture of an item of clothing on fire, such as a shirt, or hold a picture of flames up to clothing. Teach children the importance of fire safety without frightening them.

Familiarize children with various warning alarms for fire. Alarms may include loud tones, verbal warning, and flashing lights. Practice fire drills regularly (for example, monthly) and vary the practice drills so children know what to do whether they are in the classroom, on the playground, or in the restroom. Children may have difficulty following procedures during the first few emergency practices. Continue to practice the individual steps of the emergency drill, and reinforce learning through other routines and activities. Once children are familiar with the primary exit route and procedures, you can practice a second way out. Having two ways out is important in case the primary exit is blocked.

Safety guidance is most effective when teachers have appropriate expectations and when safety rules are stated in a positive manner. Explain to children that they gather to exit the classroom the same way they gather for meals, outdoor playtime, and emergency drills. Focus on one type of emergency drill at a time (for example, fire drill this week and earthquake drill another week). Through practice and routines, children are better able to follow your instruction and guidance. Evaluate each child's knowledge and skill in this area, and provide additional learning activities as needed to ensure that all children can follow emergency routines.

Other Emergency Situations

Once children understand and can demonstrate appropriate response to a fire drill, you may begin to introduce other emergency situations that require an immediate action by the children while in your program.

For example, tornadoes and other weather conditions can cause devastating damage in just a few seconds. Many local television or radio stations have meteorologists (weather forecasters) who will visit your classroom to talk with children about safety related to tornadoes and other weather conditions. First, everyone should get the warning through a National Oceanic and Atmospheric Administration (NOAA) weather radio, smartphone, or WeatherCall to a phone or cell phone. Next, know your safe place; in structured buildings, the safest area is a small room (for example, a hallway, closet, or bathroom) on the lowest floor, away from windows, and near the center of the building. Put as many walls between you and the tornado as possible. Crouch as low as possible to the floor, facing down, and cover your head with your hands. Mobile homes and metal "warehouse" type structures are not safe in severe weather. At the first warning, evacuate to a safer shelter.

Address the weather emergency or emergencies that are most likely to occur in your geographic area. It is also a good idea to address lockdown procedures in case of potentially violent situations. All staff and volunteers should be familiar with the program's written policy and procedure for emergency situations, and they should practice all drills regularly.

Regardless of the emergency, your goal is to be prepared and keep yourself and children safe. Teach children to listen and follow your instructions. With practice and a calm response, you will be more prepared in case of a true emergency.

VOCABULARY

alarm	evacuation	meteorologist	tornado
burn	exit	practice	volcano
cover	fire	roll	warning
drill	flames	route	wind
drop	flood	shelter	
emergency	heat	smoke detector	
escape	hurricane	storm	

CREATING THE ENVIRONMENT

- Check that your facility has working smoke detectors, a fire alarm system, accessible fire extinguishers, fire doors, and several exit routes. Post evacuation routes by the classroom door, and assure that all staff and volunteers are familiar with all routes.

- Familiarize children with various warning alarms. Practice emergency drills regularly.

- Carefully check the classroom and playground for fire and burn hazards. If extension cords must be used, regularly inspect them for signs of wear, and position the extension cords so children cannot pull them or trip over them. Never place an electrical cord under a rug or carpet. Cover electrical outlets when not in use.

- Carefully supervise cooking activities that require the use of electrical appliances or result in hot foods. Add props like pot holders and smoke alarms to learning centers to encourage fire safety.

- Use an early warning system for weather conditions in your area (for example, NOAA weather radio or a smartphone). Do not rely on community tornado sirens for early warning.

EVALUATION

- During role play, do children include evacuation action?
- Are children discussing fire or other emergencies?
- Can children show what to do in case of smoke or fire?
- Do children increasingly listen and follow adult instructions during emergency drills and practice activities?
- Are children increasingly initiating appropriate response to emergency drills?

CHILDREN'S ACTIVITIES

The Heat Is On

Provide something warm for children to feel and talk about. Ask them if they can remember a time when something warm felt good to them. See if they can remember a time when something was too warm (hot) and it hurt to touch it. Let them know that many various things can be too hot (including water, playground equipment in the sun, ovens, food, fire, and so on). Discuss getting burned and how to avoid it. Ask children how they think things get warm or hot. Talk about different ways to get something hot, such as plugging it in, putting it in the oven, putting it in a fire, or leaving it in the sun. Let each child select an object to take outside to put in the sun. Have children write their names on pieces of paper to be placed near or taped to their objects (help as needed). Encourage children to check on their objects throughout the day and talk about the temperature change.

❶ Safety Note: Ensure that what children feel is warm, not hot. Do not leave a heating pad plugged in or unattended. Children should wash and dry their hands before the activity. Check for appropriate temperature before initiating the outside sunning portion of this activity.

MATERIALS
- a warm object to feel (such as water, a warm hand cloth, a hot-water bottle, a heating pad, a coin in the sun, or a muffin fresh out of the oven), objects selected by children, paper, pen, and tape

OTHER IDEAS
- Invite children to feel ice cubes and a hot-water bottle, and then compare the experiences.

- Show children a variety of nonmercury thermometers (indoor, outdoor, cooking, medical, and so on), and help them read the temperature in various locations. Explain the range of temperature from cold to hot, and safety considerations.

- Add a play or real barbecue grill to the dramatic play interest area or outdoors for role play. Let children know that it heats (cooks) food and that when real ones are used, they can get too hot to touch.

- Show children a reflective emergency blanket, and discuss the properties and purposes. Place the blanket in the dramatic play interest area after the activity.

By the Light of the Fire

Introduce and play flute songs as a calming activity. Tell children that you are going to light a fire (a candle, oil lamp, or lamp with a flame-shaped bulb), and that it is important they stay behind the line you have made on the floor with tape or rope. Walk around the line, and demonstrate where children are to stay. Explain that you want to show them a flame, but they need to know that children should not start fires because it is too dangerous. After you light the fire, ask children to talk about times they have seen a fire. Ask if they have seen lighted candles at home. Ask if they have seen a fire in a fireplace or have been to a bonfire. Tell the children that some people use candles to celebrate special events. Ask if they can think of ways fire is used to help us. Help children understand that heat is used to cook and keep homes warm. Thank children for staying a safe distance from the flame, and let them know that you are going to extinguish the flame.

❗Safety Note: Be sure adequate supervision is available for this activity. Test the candle or lamp prior to the activity. A physical reminder of the boundary is important. With close guidance, children can learn appropriate behavior around fire. Exposure to planned and supervised situations gives children the opportunity to practice skills.

MATERIALS
- masking tape or rope to mark boundaries, flute music (such as from the album *Dream Catcher* by Tokeya Inajin), a candle or oil lamp

OTHER IDEAS
- Visit a candle maker to observe the process. Point out the safety precautions the artist takes.

- Visit a glassblower to see the creations and watch how flames are used for this art. Point out the safety precautions the artist takes.

- Read the following books or others that feature candles, and discuss how candles are used in tradition and celebration: *Lights of Winter: Winter Celebrations around the World* by Heather Conrad, *Nathan Blows Out the Hanukkah Candles* by Tami Lehman-Wilzig, *One Candle* by Eve Bunting, *Candle Carrie the Birthday Fairy* by Joanne Gazzal, *Light Your Candle* by Carl Sommer. Talk with children about how each family has their own beliefs and ways of celebrating.

■ Read selected sections and discuss *The Charcoal Forest: How Fire Helps Animals & Plants* by Beth A. Peluso. Help

children understand that while the forest fire caused damage to the trees and may have harmed and relocated some animals, some good for the earth also resulted from it.

Flames

Show children a rolling pin and how it works. See how many other things they can find in the classroom or on the playground that roll, such as balls, tires, cans, and bottles. Ask for volunteers to roll their bodies. Let all the children who are interested show you how they can roll. Help those who have difficulty. Show children pictures or photographs of clothes (not people) that are on fire and tell the children that if the clothes they are wearing ever catch on fire, they should "Stop, drop, and roll" like a rolling pin. Show them how to do this as you say it. Have them practice chanting it with you. Follow up at later times to help them remember.

MATERIALS
- a rolling pin, a large open space to practice rolling, pictures or photographs of clothes (not people) on fire

OTHER IDEAS
- Encourage children to find something in the room that rolls and to demonstrate it for the other children. End the activity with everyone practicing their "Stop, drop, and roll" movements.

- Provide playdough and a variety of rolling pins for children to use and discuss. Remind children about how they should "Stop, drop, and roll" if the clothes they are wearing ever catch on fire.

- Let children roll on a variety of surfaces, such as grass, carpet, pillows, and tile. Discuss how each surface feels and the importance of using "Stop, drop, and roll" if their clothes catch on fire.

- Incorporate "Stop, drop, and roll" into traditional games like Simon Says.

Smoke

Ask children to hold a parachute or bedsheet "up high," "in the middle," and "down low." Repeat these actions a few times. Place a ball on the parachute for children to roll from side to side. Roll a ball under the parachute to a child, and then let several children roll the ball under the parachute. Hold the parachute "at medium" and ask for volunteers to take the ball and crawl under the parachute to the other side. Encourage each child to try crawling under the parachute, with or without the ball, and with or without a classmate. Help the children see the difference between rolling and crawling. After the children have all had a turn, have them sit with you so you can show them photographs of smoke. Invite them to discuss the photos. Tell them that in case of smoke (caused by a fire and not a candle or a tobacco product), they need to "Get low and go, go, go!" Have children chant "Get low and go, go, go!" with you. Let the children practice crawling under the parachute again, pretending that it is smoke.

MATERIALS
- a parachute, balls, and photographs of smoke

OTHER IDEAS

- Provide a box open at both ends and large enough for children to crawl through. Let children glue gray tissue paper to the "ceiling" of the box, creating a smoky atmosphere. Once the tissue paper has dried, encourage children to crawl through the box while chanting "Get low and go, go, go!"

- Play the song "Limbo Rock" by one of many artists, such as Samuel E. Wright or Dora the Explorer, and teach the children how to play a game of limbo, ending up with them crawling under the obstacle (string, stick, human bridge) to practice "Get low and go, go, go!"

- Provide several smoke alarms for children to examine and let them hear the alarm sound. Talk about how the sound can help wake people who are sleeping or alert them if they are busy working or playing. Explain that smoke alarms sounding means people should evacuate, and describe evacuation. Go on a smoke alarm walk through the facility to look for smoke alarms.

- Read and discuss *"Fire! Fire!" Said Mrs. McGuire* by Bill Martin Jr.

Earth, Water, and Wind

Provide dishpans, each filled with a different soil type to examine. Ask the children to describe the textures, smells, and appearances. Let children measure the soils and weigh the containers. See if they know of any other words people use to describe soil (earth, dirt, clay, sand, land, crust, ground, and so on). Ask children what things use soil, and encourage them to consider plants, animals, people, and structures. Let children add toy animals, plants, people, and structures to the soils. Tell them that in some places at some times the ground moves for a few seconds, and ask what they think happens to the animals, plants, people, and buildings when that happens. Allow children to shake the containers of soil and observe. Let children know that when the earth moves, it is called an earthquake and that it is an emergency. Everyone should "Drop, cover, and hold on!" in an earthquake. Encourage the children to practice dropping to the floor, taking cover under a table, and holding on while they chant "Drop, cover, and hold on!"

❗Safety Note: Check soil in advance for any harmful material such as broken glass or animal droppings.

MATERIALS

- dishpans of various soil types (such as sand, clay, topsoil, and so on), a ruler, a scale, and toys (for example, plants, animals, people, and structures)

OTHER IDEAS

- Using a dishpan with one inch of soil, involve children in inserting upside-down bottle caps in the soil to represent lakes. Ask what they think will happen when the lakes get full of water. Pour water slowly, and encourage children to watch for the overflow. Let them take turns gently feeling the soil as it absorbs water. Keep pouring until there is more water than soil. Explain briefly that when it rains too fast and for too long, water overflows and causes a flood, which is an emergency. Let children know that during a flood people should "Get to higher ground" and stay out of the water. Take a walk, and look for higher ground (upstairs, on hills, at the top of steps).

- Demonstrate what an erupting volcano looks like. Put two tablespoons of baking soda in a plastic bottle, replace the lid, and put the bottle on a tray to catch the mess.

Engage children in building a mud mountain to cover all but the lid of the bottle. Once the mountain is dry, gather children, and remove the bottle lid before pouring a cup of vinegar with red food coloring into the bottle. Watch for the eruption—it will be fast but can be repeated. Let children know that volcanoes are caused when the hot core in the center of the earth moves to the top and then begins to pour out. Assure them that this does not happen often or in many places. Let children know if they live far from potentially active volcanoes. Explain that when a volcano erupts, it is an emergency, and people need to get away from it because it is hot and the lava flow may move fast. Remind them that adults should be able to help them move to safety.

■ Show children a tornado in a 2 liter bottle. Fill one bottle over half full of water and add metallic confetti, glitter, or food coloring to enhance the visual aspects of the activity. Place the empty bottle on top of the other bottle and fasten them together with the commercial Tornado Tube or by creating your own connection. For alternatives to the inexpensive Tornado Tube, use a circular object with a hole in the center smaller than the bottle opening. Place the circular object, such as a washer, tubing, or pipe, between the bottles and wrap tightly with duct tape. Once the tornado in a bottle is prepared, turn it so that the water is on top and twist in a circular motion until a funnel forms. Let children know that a funnel like that in the sky is called a tornado and that it is a column of wind rotating during a thunderstorm. Make sure children know that tornadoes are emergencies and that when one occurs, people should "take shelter" in a basement or a room with no windows. Show them how to use their hands to cover their heads. End the activity by showing children where the tornado shelter is in the building and letting them practice protecting their heads.

■ Read and discuss one of these or other books on hurricanes: *Hurricane* by David Wiesner; *Two Bobbies: A True Story of Hurricane Katrina, Friendship, and Survival* by Kirby Larson and Mary Nethery; or *Hurricane!* by Jonathan London.

Practice for Emergencies

Show children photographs or a video clip of building fires or wildfires, and tell them that sometimes fire gets too big and is hard to stop. Explain that while firefighters work to stop the fire, everyone else needs to get away from the fire so they will be safe. Tell children that we need to practice how to get away from a fire so we are ready if there is one. Let children hear and see a variety of alarms (sirens, visual signaling equipment, bells, and so on), including the ones sounded at your program for fire and tornado drills. Announce that when they hear a sound like one of these, they should stop playing immediately (freeze) and listen for directions from the teachers. Follow up by having a practice drill. Repeat for tornadoes and other likely emergencies in your area.

MATERIALS

- photographs or video clips of fire, a viewing device for the video, and several working alarms with different sounds (Local emergency services or vendors may be able to provide samples. Sound clips are also available online—type "sound clip of sirens" into an online search engine.)

OTHER IDEAS

- Show children an exit sign, and explain what it is. Discuss how exit signs are located near doors that lead outside. Remind children that during a fire drill, everyone goes outside as quickly as it is safe to go. Take a walk to look for exit signs and see where all exits lead. Help children understand that exit signs may look different (they may be made of metal or paper, for example), but that all have the same letters: EXIT (or alternate language). Point out that windows, as well as doors, lead outside, and practice exiting windows. Repeat the activity using a tornado shelter sign, and remind children that during tornadoes, the safe place is indoors, not out.

- Arrange for children to watch an older class practicing a fire drill, and point out what the children are doing that you want your class to do during their drill. Discuss their observations, and then practice a fire drill with the group. Repeat with a tornado drill.

  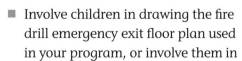

- Involve children in drawing the fire drill emergency exit floor plan used in your program, or involve them in coloring the preferred escape path on an existing program floor plan. Let each child hold a copy of the floor plan, and walk the route as a group, pausing to help them see where they are on the map and in the building. Repeat the walk at other times, allowing various children to lead the way. Try the activity using the tornado drill route.

■ Play and sing the song "Fire Drill" by Justin Roberts.

FAMILY INFORMATION

MY RULES FOR EMERGENCIES!

Many types of emergencies can occur at home. One of the most common emergencies is fire. In just thirty seconds, a small flame from a dropped match can become a fire burning out of control. The smoke and heat can be deadly. If your smoke detector alarm sounds, you may have less than two minutes to get out of the house!

Install smoke detectors on the ceiling or high on the wall on each floor in your home. Place detectors close to bedrooms and at the top of stairs. Test the smoke detectors monthly. If the smoke detectors use batteries, change the batteries twice each year. Let children help you test the smoke detector so they know the alarm sound.

Teach your child to stay safe:

- If you see or smell smoke, or the alarm sounds, get out of the house!

- "Stop, drop, and roll" if your clothes catch on fire.

- If you see or smell smoke, "Get low and go, go, go!"

GO TO THE MEETING PLACE

Show your child how to get out of the house. This may mean going out a window. Practice opening a locked window. Show your child how to push out a screen. If the window is a few feet above the ground, show your child how to hang from his or her hands and drop to the ground.

Choose a safe meeting place outside where everyone should go.

FAMILY ACTIVITY

Ask your child what she or he thinks is happening in the picture below while coloring it. Talk with your child about what to do at home in an emergency such as a fire, flood, tornado, or earthquake.

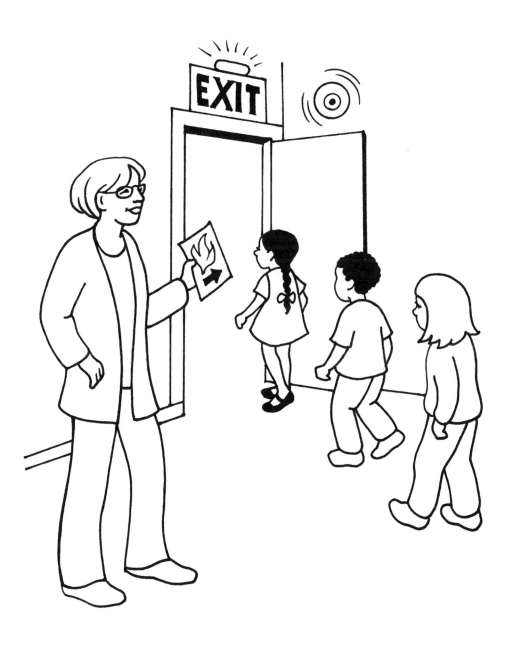

4

I Want to Help, Not Hurt!

LEARNING OBJECTIVES

- Children will identify peaceful ways to resolve conflict.
- Children will recognize weapons (including knives).
- Children will communicate what to do if they find a weapon.

Violence and the availability of weapons comprise an issue that many young children face in our society. Too often children do not comprehend the difference between a toy and a real gun. They may play with a "toy" weapon, only to learn too late that it is real.

Children may be exposed to weapons in a variety of ways. They may come in contact with military and law enforcement personnel and hunters who use guns as tools of their work. Some adults enjoy collecting guns, knives, and other weapons. Help children understand that it is not wrong for an adult to own a weapon, but that children and adults can be hurt by weapons if they are not used safely. Children often watch television programs and movies that show weapons being used, and they may see weapons in their home, at a friend's home, or in the community. Unfortunately, some children may encounter individuals who intend to hurt others, including through domestic violence. However, care should be taken not to frighten children unnecessarily or use negative labels, such as "bad guys," when referring to people who carry or use weapons.

For children to avoid potential hazards, they must first recognize the hazard. Depending on the community or culture, children may be exposed to BB guns, hunting rifles, knives, swords, or military weapons, such as grenades. Determine what weapons (for example, rifles, handguns, knives, bows and arrows) are prevalent in your community, and what dangers young children may face (for example, hunting incidents, finding a gun in a closet or on a playground, drive-by shooting, or gang violence). Know and understand your community and potential risks. Engage parents and families in this discussion.

Provide children with factual information regarding weapons and what they should do if they find one. If children find a weapon, they should not touch it. They should tell an adult, lead the adult to the location, and point to (not touch) the weapon.

VOCABULARY

accident	collector	hurt	rifle
arrow	conflict	kind	soldier
bow	cut	knife	sword
cannon	dynamite	military	weapon
carve	gun	peaceful	
chef	hand grenade	police	
choose	hunter	resolution	

CREATING THE ENVIRONMENT

■ Show children photographs or replicas of weapons in small-group discussions, but do not leave items out for free play or learning-center time. Weapons, including replicas or photographs of weapons, are not appropriate for school use except when you are teaching about safety.

■ When using replicas as a teaching tool, show them to the children but do not allow them to touch the replicas. This reinforces the idea that children should not touch weapons.

EVALUATION

■ Do children talk about and ask questions regarding weapons, including those they may have seen (for example, at home, on television, in a book)?

■ Can children demonstrate what to do if they find a weapon (for example, on a playground, in their home)?

■ During role play, can children communicate what to do if they find a weapon (for example, on a playground)?

■ During guided activities, can children demonstrate understanding that they should not touch knives, except with adult supervision (that is, during cooking activities)?

■ Are children discussing or displaying peaceful resolutions to conflicts?

CHILDREN'S ACTIVITIES

Clap and Stomp

Begin clapping your hands. Invite children to clap along with you. Start stomping your feet, and encourage children to stomp. Introduce fast and lively music to encourage children's dancing and clapping. After the music, ask children for words that describe what they were doing. Accept general answers such as dancing or moving. Prompt children to describe more specifically what they were doing with their hands and their feet to focus them on clapping (or slapping their hands together) and stomping. Explain that although this activity was fun and no one was hurt, sometimes slapping hands and stomping feet hurt. If they slap their own hands together too hard or stomp their own feet on the floor too roughly, it could hurt. Ask children to recall any time when they have seen people or characters on a television show hit or kick something or someone and something broke or it looked like someone got hurt. Encourage them to talk about things they can do instead of hitting or kicking when they are mad or upset. Examples may include using words to express their feelings, asking an adult for help, turning away and finding something else fun to do, or taking deep breaths to calm down. Reassure children who are fearful.

MATERIALS
■ dancing music and a music player

OTHER IDEAS

■ Visit or invite a conflict resolution counselor or peace advocate to tell about his job and ideas for using peaceful resolutions.

■ Have children make several handprints using tempera paint, and assist as needed to write their name on each. Explain that all but one of their handprints will be put into the Kind Hands Box, which they can help decorate. Tell them that when someone does something kind for them, they should get a handprint of that child out of the box (or ask the teacher to help them get it) and post the hand on the special Kind Hands Bulletin Board. If some children are not recognized on the bulletin board, ask a child to do something helpful and then post the child's hand. Periodically, review the hands on the bulletin board and what kindness each child has shown.

▪ Play "Clap Your Hands" by Tickle Tune Typhoon. Follow up by discussing with children harmful and helpful things they can do with their hands.

▪ Reinforce how stomping and clapping can be a fun activity or it can be hurtful if someone is angry or directs the action toward others. Play "Stomp and Clap" by the Learning Station.

Beat the Drum

Invite children to select various rhythm band instruments to play as they march to music. After children have returned their instruments, ask them to describe what they were doing. Prompt children to describe the activity with words like *hit* and *shake*. Tell children that you think it is fun to play instruments by hitting and shaking them. Ask what they think about using the instruments to hit someone. Tell them that objects used to hurt people are called *weapons*, and ask if they have heard the word. Explain that although someone could hit with a musical instrument, it is not called a weapon unless it is being used in that way. Remind them that it is important to find peaceful ways to work out differences instead of hitting.

MATERIALS
- marching music, a music player, and rhythm instruments (such as drums, rhythm sticks, tambourines, cymbals, bells, and so on)

OTHER IDEAS

- Provide supplies, and let children create musical instruments that require hitting and shaking to play. Discuss hitting and shaking in a variety of situations, like making music rather than responding angrily.

- Play music, and lead the children through shaking their various body parts. Discuss the difference between shaking your own body part and shaking someone else's.

- Play and listen to "Peace Will Come" and "I'd Rather Be Singing" by Grenadilla. Talk with the children about what they think each song means.

- Play and listen to the words of "Stop, Think, Choose" and "Get Along" by Steve Couch. Talk with children about choices they have when they are angry. Help them identify a variety of acceptable actions, such as using words to express their feelings, requesting help from an adult, turning and finding something else fun, or taking deep breaths to calm down.

Picturing Weapons

Show children pictures or photographs of weapons (guns, knives, swords, bows and arrows, nunchucks, and so on) and ask them to tell you what they know about them. Explain that you are showing them pictures to be sure they know what weapons look like. Tell them they should not touch a weapon if they see one, but they should tell an adult. Explain that they could get hurt or hurt someone else without meaning to if they pick up a weapon. Ask them to name some adults they could tell if they find a weapon. Let the children look for pictures of weapons in magazines and cut or tear them out. Help the children make puzzles by pasting the pictures onto cardboard and then cutting them into puzzle pieces. As children make their puzzles, point out the differences in the guns. Stress that they should not touch guns and they should tell an adult if they see a weapon.

MATERIALS

- pictures or photographs of weapons—select ones based on your local community and the backgrounds of the children served, and focus on those the children are most likely to encounter; magazines, catalogs, cardboard, paste or glue, scissors, and an envelope for storing puzzle pieces

OTHER IDEAS

- Visit a store that sells weapons, and help children recognize that weapons can look a variety of ways. For example, guns may be a rifle or handgun, and knives may be a dagger, survival tool, or pocketknife.

- Visit a store that sells gun cabinets and knife cases for safe storage. Ask the store clerk to show the safety features of selected products and talk about the importance of weapons being locked.

- Read and discuss *True Blue* by Joan Elste. Summarize and explain content as appropriate for the age of the children served. Objectively introduce unfamiliar terms, such as *hunters* or *poachers*.

- Read and discuss *There's a Nightmare in My Closet* by Mercer Mayer. After examining the illustrations, talk with children about the difference between toy guns and real guns, and explain that it is sometimes difficult to tell the difference.

Shout It Loud!

Show children pictures and photographs of weapons, one at a time. After you show each picture, ask the children what it is and what they should do if they find one like it. Prompt the children with questions until they say something like, "Do not touch a weapon" or "Go tell an adult." Repeat those phrases back to them and tell them that rule number one is "Do not touch a weapon," and rule number two is "Go tell an adult." Invite the children to say rule number one with you louder, then louder, and then even louder. Repeat with rule number two. Chant the rules with the children using a loud tone then a low tone. Say them fast and say them slowly. Say the rules with the children standing up, sitting down, lying on the floor, and standing on one foot. Chant the rules using languages other than English.

MATERIALS

■ pictures or photographs of weapons

OTHER IDEAS

■ Provide art materials, and assist each child in creating a "Rules for Weapons" poster that contains the two rules and their illustrations. Write the rules for children to see and copy, or provide copies of the rules printed in large text that they can glue to their poster and draw illustrations around. Display posters for a few days, and then encourage children to take them home.

■ Create an enlarged and laminated teacher-made "Rules for Weapons" poster, and cut it into pieces for a floor jigsaw puzzle.

■ Assist children in creating a class video of the two rules for weapons. Use replicas of weapons, and have children act out finding one, leaving it alone, and going to tell an adult. Repeat the scene several times with the weapon replica in various places and with all children involved in the video in some way.

■ Create a puppet show with children that will allow them to practice saying the two rules for weapons. One puppet can be a teacher asking other puppets that are children what they should do if they find a gun (or a knife or another weapon).

Helpful Ways

Show children pictures or photographs of tools that are also real or potential weapons, and ask for ways that these tools (weapons) are used that might be helpful. Examples might include the following: a knife is used to cut food, a knife is used to carve wood, a gun is used by a police officer or soldier to help keep us safe, a gun or a bow and arrow are used to hunt animals for food, dynamite is used to clear rock for a new road, a cannon is used at football games to celebrate points made. During conversation, point out that although adults may use the tools in useful ways, most of them are not meant for young children to use. Explain that classroom tools such as woodworking and cooking tools are to be used with adult permission and supervision. Remind them not to touch a tool that can hurt or any other weapon and to tell an adult if they see one.

MATERIALS

- pictures of tools that are real or potential weapons mounted on cardboard

OTHER IDEAS

- Visit or invite soldiers or police officers to talk about how they use weapons to keep us safe and about safety precautions they take with their weapons.

- Visit or invite someone who hunts animals for food, and ask the visitor to talk about the importance of feeding her family and about safety precautions she takes with her weapon.

- Visit or invite a wood-carver or someone who whittles to demonstrate his craft and to discuss the proper care and storage of his tools to avoid accidents.

- Visit or invite a chef to talk about the use of knives in food preparation, to demonstrate her trade, and to discuss proper care and storage of her tools to avoid accidents.

No Flying Weapon

Tell children that adults have rules to follow too. Adults are not allowed to take weapons some places, such as on airplanes, unless they are police officers. Hold up a toy airplane, and explain that before you ride on an airplane, you must go through a metal detector so guards can check for weapons. Explain that going through the security at the airport is just like walking through a door and does not hurt. If possible, arrange a field trip with security officials at the local airport, and announce that you will be visiting the airport to see a metal detector in use. Ask a security worker to explain how his job helps keep people safe.

MATERIALS
- a toy airplane

OTHER IDEAS

- After the airport trip or looking at a video clip of people going through a metal detector, help children develop a replica of a metal detector for their use in role play.

  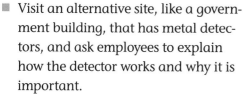

- Visit an alternative site, like a government building, that has metal detectors, and ask employees to explain how the detector works and why it is important.

- Invite a lawyer or police officer to visit and explain the rules adults must follow regarding weapons, such as needing a license to carry them.

- Take a walk, and look for signs that show rules that adults must follow, such as "No weapons allowed."

FAMILY INFORMATION

I WANT TO HELP, NOT HURT!

Violence and the availability of weapons have created an issue that many young children face in our society. Children may find weapons at home, at a friend's house, or even on a playground. In communities near military bases, children may find explosives, such as hand grenades.

Children may play with what they think is a toy gun or hand grenade, only to learn too late that it is real. Teach your child that all weapons should be considered real and should not be touched. This includes guns, military weapons, hunting knives, bows and arrows, mace and pepper spray, and even BB guns.

Explain to children that it may be okay for adults to own weapons, but children can be hurt by weapons if they are not used safely.

WHAT TO DO

The rule is "Don't touch a weapon!" Teach your child that if he or she finds a weapon, she or he should not touch it and should go tell an adult, lead the adult to the location, and point to (not touch) the weapon.

If you have weapons in your home, store them in a locked cabinet or closet, and store ammunition separately. You may want to find out if there are weapons in other homes your child visits.

FAMILY ACTIVITY

Begin a discussion about what is happening in the picture. Consider discussing with your child what you would like your child to do when he or she gets mad at someone, what to do if she or he sees someone hurting or bullying someone else, and what to do if he or she sees someone with a weapon or finds a knife, gun, or other weapon that could be used to hurt someone. Be sure to answer questions such as where to go and who to seek help from.

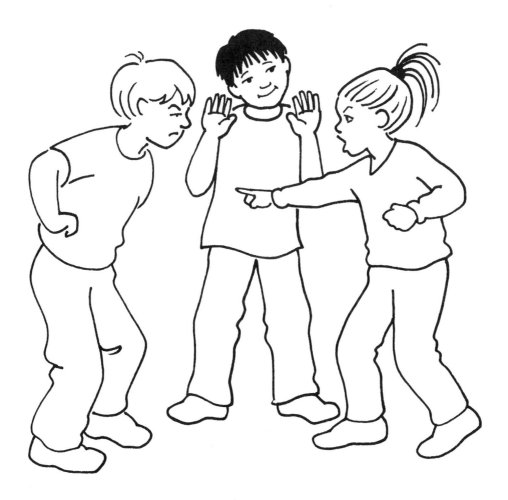

Violence is not the answer!

What Goes between My Lips and into My Mouth

LEARNING OBJECTIVES

- Children will identify items as food or nonfood.
- Children will state what might happen if nonfood items are put into their mouths.
- Children will communicate why they should ask an adult before eating or drinking something unfamiliar, even if it looks like food.

Children, especially young children, often explore and learn about new items by putting them in their mouths. Older children may chew on items (for example, pencils) or put objects in their mouths out of habit. Adult should create an environment that is as safe as possible and should help children recognize the danger of putting nonfood items in their mouths.

Be aware of the dangers of potentially toxic substances in the school environment. Some substances, such as toilet cleaner and dishwasher detergent, may contain corrosive chemicals that severely burn the mouth, throat, and stomach in just a few seconds. Products containing petroleum, such as gasoline or turpentine, can cause damage if swallowed or inhaled. Plants are among the most common household substances that children ingest—and many common ones are poisonous.

Toxic substances, such as sanitizing materials, pesticides, detergents, and rubber cement, must be stored in the original labeled container. Keep these substances out of children's sight, out of reach, and in a locked cabinet, preferably in a room or area of the facility inaccessible to children. Toxic items should never be stored near food or medications.

Items for personal use, such as medication, cosmetics, hand sanitizer, and shampoos, can be potentially toxic for young children. Store these products out of children's sight and reach, and allow use only with adult supervision.

All plants in areas accessible to children, both indoors and outdoors, must be nonpoisonous. Young children have difficulty differentiating between berries that we eat, such as blackberries or blueberries, and berries that are toxic, such as those on holly bushes and mistletoe. Learn the names of plants in your outdoor area, and then check with the regional Poison Center for information on toxicity. You can reach your local poison center by calling 1-800-222-1222.

Choking is a hazard for young children because they often put toys and other items in their mouths. Check all toys for small, broken, or removable parts. Never allow latex balloons in the children's environment. Latex balloons are one of the leading choking hazards for both young and older children. Mylar balloons are much safer.

Children—and adults—may also choke on food items; supervise so children do not run, jump, or play actively with food, gum, or candy in their mouths. Foods that are hard or round, such as hot dogs, hard candy, grapes, nuts, and popcorn, are prime choking culprits. Sticky foods, such as a spoonful of peanut butter, marshmallows, or raisins, can block a child's air passage. Meats and tough foods are difficult for young children to chew since they may not have their back teeth or developed chewing skills. Teach children to enjoy foods by chewing slowly and thoroughly.

Check with your area children's hospital or pediatric clinic for more information on preventing choking, and always have at least one person trained in first aid and CPR available, including on field trips.

VOCABULARY

berries	contaminated	nonfood	strangle
boil	danger	nuts	swallow
burn	dirty	pesticide	toxic
caution	edible	plant	venomous
choke	impure	poison	
clean	infected	polluted	
cleaner	locked	raw	

CREATING THE ENVIRONMENT

- Keep all potentially toxic items in a locked cabinet: cleaning solutions, bleach and other disinfectants, rubber cement, medications, and aerosols.

- Read labels; make sure all art and craft supplies are nontoxic.

- Identify plants in your indoor and outdoor environment. Remove potentially toxic plants from indoors and outdoors, if possible.

- Prepare foods served to children in a way that prevents choking, such as cutting hot dogs into small squares (not circles), cutting raw vegetables into skinny strips rather than chunks, separating raisins, and serving only a thin layer of peanut butter on crackers.

- Post the National Capital Poison Center number in the classroom and near all telephones: 1-800-222-1222.

- Train staff members in first aid, choking response, and CPR.

- Check toys for broken or small parts.

EVALUATION

- Can children talk about the effects of poison?

- Do children sort food and nonfood items during play?

- Can children communicate why they should ask an adult before eating or drinking an unfamiliar item?

- During outdoor activities (for example, nature walks), can children communicate that it is unsafe to put unidentified berries, nuts, or other items in their mouths?

- Do children discuss why nonfood items might cause choking?

CHILDREN'S ACTIVITIES

Tabletop

Get input from families, and gather a diverse sampling of items other than food that might be on a dinner table. Cover the items with a tablecloth. Tell children to name things that might be on a table where people eat. Draw a line down the middle of a piece of chart paper, and write *food* at the top on one side, and *not food* on the other. As children name things, ask them to specify if they are or are not food. Once they have shared all their ideas, remove the tablecloth. Ask the children what each of the nonfood items is, and add to the list any that were not included originally. Count with the children all of the items on the tabletop, count the items on both sides of the list, and talk about which is the largest number. Point out that items that are not food should not be eaten, even if they are on the food table. Hold up some of the items, and ask children what they think might happen if they tried to eat them. Answers may include breaking teeth, choking, getting sick, and so on.

MATERIALS
- various nonfood items associated with eating (such as a tablecloth, candlesticks, place mats of various materials, place cards, a flower arrangement, napkins, various dishes, eating utensils, confetti, salt and pepper shakers, and decorations), a tablecloth, a marker, and chart paper

OTHER IDEAS
- Play, sing, and discuss the song "Koala Bear Diner" by Justin Roberts. Talk about how koalas and people eat different things.

- Invite families of the enrolled children to set up a table display showing how their dinner table looks for special occasions or daily meals. Pictures and photographs can be used to represent the food. Encourage families to tell short stories about the things on their table.

- Involve children in creating nonfood items that go on tabletops during meals, such as place mats, table skirts, table runners, confetti, coasters, centerpieces, place cards, napkin rings, and so on, and use them during mealtimes, making the environment pleasant and taking the opportunity to reinforce that children should not put nonfood items into their mouths.

■ Read and discuss *Feathers for Lunch* by Lois Ehlert. Ask children what they think might happen if people ate feathers for lunch.

Swallowing Flies

Read *There Was an Old Lady Who Swallowed a Fly* by Simms Taback, and discuss the many things the woman ate. Engage children in chanting the repetitive sections, and enjoy the humor with them. Then help children analyze the potential consequences of people really eating the things the old lady swallowed.

MATERIALS

■ a copy of *There Was an Old Lady Who Swallowed a Fly* by Simms Taback

OTHER IDEAS

■ Read, discuss, and compare other versions of *There Was an Old Lady Who Swallowed a Fly.* Process with children any differences in the things the lady swallowed, the style of the book, and the authors and illustrators.

■ Read and discuss *There Was an Old Lady Who Swallowed a Shell!* by Lucille Colandro. Ask children which of the things the old lady swallowed would be safe for people to eat and which would not be. Point out that a swimming fish may not be safe to eat but that people do eat fish after they are prepared.

■ Ask each child to get something from the room that the "Old Lady" could swallow. Retell the story using the children's objects. Then ask each child to name something the "Old Lady" could swallow that would be safe for her to eat, and retell the story using the safe recommendations of the child.

■ Talk about the things the "Old Lady" swallowed that could have been poisonous. Teach the children the Poison Prevention Jingles from the National Capital Poison Center at www.poison.org/jingle, or lead them in making up their own jingles about what to do if someone is poisoned.

Furry Critter Food

Put small amounts of different dry pet food into bowls. Let children feel and smell the food and guess what it is. Ask children to describe what they see, feel, and smell. Encourage them to compare the contents of each bowl to the others. Ask questions like "Which is softer?" and "Which is larger?" Show children the original containers, and read the ingredients for them. Let them see if they can match the containers to the food. Invite them to tell about any pets they have fed and how they knew what, how much, and when to feed them. After the stories, reinforce that pet food is for pets and not for people. Although it is food, it is not food for people to eat—consider donating the pet food to an animal rescue organization. If children show interest in what other animals eat, follow up by helping them to investigate.

❗ Safety Note: Children need to wash their hands after handling pet food.

MATERIALS
- a variety of dry pet food (including dog food, cat food, fish food, and hamster food) and the containers they come in

OTHER IDEAS
- Encourage children to create posters about pet food using the food itself, containers, and other art supplies. Help the children include on their poster the message that pet food is for pets, not people.

- Invite a veterinarian, pet trainer, or pet owner to talk with the children about the importance of nutrition for pets, how often pets should eat, and how much pets should eat. Remind children that both pets and people need nutritious foods, but they need different foods.

- Get a classroom pet, visiting or long-term, and do research with the children on what and how to feed the pet. Engage children in the feeding and tracking of its meals on a chart.

- Visit a pet supply store to learn about feeding pets, pet food, and pet food dishes and water bottles.

Berry Patch

Read *Blueberries for Sal* by Robert McCloskey, and talk about the story. Have children wash their hands and help prepare blueberry muffins (make blueberry pancakes on an electric griddle if you do not have access to an oven). Tell the children that some berries can be safely eaten and are good for them, but others are poisonous, so they should never eat berries they find on a plant or the ground until they check with an adult. Explain that knowing they should not eat the table decorations or pet food is pretty easy, but knowing which berries are safe to eat is harder because poisonous ones may look just like ones that are safe to eat.

MATERIALS

- *Blueberries for Sal* by Robert McCloskey, blueberry muffin mix with canned blueberries, ingredients noted on box, muffin pan, bowl, spoon, can opener, and an oven

OTHER IDEAS

- Serve blueberries in cereal, in pancakes, in a smoothie, on ice cream, alone, or in other recipes besides blueberry muffins. Involve children in food planning and preparation. Remind children that the blueberries served are safe for them, but that they should never pick and eat berries outside unless an adult says the berries are safe.

- Have a berry-tasting party and serve a wide range of berries for children to taste. Try blueberries, strawberries, raspberries, blackberries, cherries, goji berries, acai berries, bilberries (huckleberries), and more. Reassure children that the berries served are safe, but that they should not pick berries without an adult approving them. Remember that children have more taste buds and foods have a stronger taste to them. Be patient if they are not interested in tasting or do not like some of the berries.

- Visit a berry farm and pick berries. Show children how to pick, and assure them that these berries are safe. Remind them that they should always check with an adult before picking berries. As a follow-up or alternative to visiting a berry farm, plant some edible berries with the children, and encourage them to be involved in the ongoing care, monitoring, and harvesting.

■ Show children a variety of mushrooms from the grocery or a garden. Explain that like berries, some mushrooms are safe to eat and some are not. Have the children wash their hands, and encourage them to examine the mushrooms through looking, touching, smelling, and tasting.

Assure the children that these mushrooms are safe, but that they should not eat mushrooms they find growing outside. Take a mushroom walk to look for ones growing that children should not eat.

Water Walk

Select a nature site that is near water and good for walking, or prepare the program grounds with water features for a walk. Provide the children with individual water bottles half filled with water, and help them put their names on them. Inform children that they are going on a nature walk to see what water they can find. Tell them that they are to carry their water bottles with them because the water they find will not be safe for drinking. Remind them that they are to drink only from their own bottle. Invite them to take paper and pencils to sketch what they see. If appropriate, carry a container with paper, pencils, a tape measure, a camera, magnifying glasses, additional safe drinking water to add to the children's bottles, and any other tools to enhance the walk. Look for puddles, streams, ponds, rivers, water dishes for pets, birdbaths, water fountains, or any other water. Discuss each formation of water you discover, and reinforce that it is not water for people to drink, it could make people sick if they did.

❗Safety Note: Young children can drown in only inches of water. Take precautions by visiting the site first to ensure paths are far enough from water sources. Also ensure that enough adults are available for supervision.

MATERIALS
- individual water bottle for each child, marker for labeling bottles, paper, pencils, a tape measure, a camera, magnifying glasses, and formations of water (natural or placed)

OTHER IDEAS
- Let children fill ice cube trays or other containers with tap water. Involve children in placing the trays and containers in a freezer and checking their progress as they change from liquid to solid. Serve the ice in water or another drink, and talk about how the water changed. Explain that the water used to make the ice was clean water, but that ice made from dirty water is dirty ice and unsafe to use.

- Explain that tap water may come from rivers, lakes, streams, springs, ponds, or underground water, but that it is treated to clean it and tested to be sure it is safe. Visit a water treatment plant, view a video clip of one, or invite someone who works at one to briefly explain the process to the children.

■ Show children water filters that are used in homes, and explain how they block out germs. Let children use a colander to sift dirt with small rocks. Compare the dirt to the water, and the rocks to germs that cannot get through filters.

■ Explain that hikers and campers who travel by foot into the woods or desert may not be able to carry enough water with them and must find ways to clean the water they can find. Tell them that one way to clean water is to boil it for one to three minutes. If the environment allows, show children what boiling water looks like, and point out the steam. Alternatively, provide a video clip of boiling water. Let the children use a stopwatch to see how long one minute is. Follow up by explaining that in some countries the government requires that water be cleaned for people before it is used, but in other countries individual families must boil their own water. Let children know about the water purification system where they live.

Kitchen Cabinets

Include children in gathering kitchen supplies from the dramatic play area, and place them on a tablecloth to examine. Have children group the items many different ways (sequenced by size, foods they like and ones they do not, food they have at home and food they do not have at home, and so on). Ask what else they think their family keeps in the kitchen cabinets. Show them some empty containers of poisonous products that are typically kept in kitchens. Explain that the containers have useful ingredients for killing germs, but that if eaten, they are poisonous. Explain that poisons can make them sick if they eat or drink them, and that some can burn their skin and make it hurt. Encourage children to talk to an adult about poisons in their home since it is not always easy to tell what is and is not poisonous. Ask children to return supplies to the dramatic play area. Immediately remove all poison containers used in the activity.

❶ Safety Note: Even empty poison containers can be extremely dangerous, especially drain cleaner and dishwasher detergent containers. Clean the outside of containers in advance, glue the tops closed, and keep them stored in a locked cabinet. Immediately after the activity, remove containers from children's reach.

MATERIALS

- kitchen supplies from the dramatic play area, tablecloth, and empty containers of common poisonous household products (such as a dishwasher detergent container, a mouse bait box, a can of rust remover, a drain opener bottle, a bug spray can, or a bleach bottle)

OTHER IDEAS

- Provide labels from poison containers, and involve children in making a class display. Discuss the dangers, and remind children that they should not touch these products if they see them somewhere and that they should ask an adult if they are not sure what something is.

- Visit a store to look for products that may be poisonous, and talk about how it is hard to tell if something is a poison.

- Invite a health professional to explain what happens to someone's body when it is poisoned. Inform the professional of the age of the children, and encourage him to be honest and provide basic information that is not graphic enough to frighten children.

■ Print and post or project free poison control prevention posters to review with the children from sites such as www.poison.org/prevent/posters .asp or www.epa.gov/oppfead1 /Publications/lockitup-poster.pdf. Select posters to include on the family bulletin board or to send home.

FAMILY INFORMATION

WHAT GOES BETWEEN MY LIPS AND INTO MY MOUTH

Cleaning supplies, bleach, makeup, shampoo, insecticides, and many other products typically found in the home can be poisonous if swallowed. For example, cleaners such as dishwasher detergent, toilet cleaner, and drain cleaner can cause severe burns in the mouth, throat, and stomach.

Keep all cleaning supplies, insecticides, chemicals, and other products in the original containers. After using these products, secure the tops, and store them out of sight and out of children's reach. Never store potentially toxic products on shelves or in cabinets where children can reach them, even if you have safety latches.

KEEP MEDICINES OUT OF SIGHT AND OUT OF REACH

Medicines, vitamins, and herbal products can be harmful if taken inappropriately. Many products are colorful and may even taste good to children. Store these products in their original labeled containers and in locked cabinets.

PLANT SAFETY

Many plants are poisonous. Some cause swelling in the mouth and breathing problems. Many wild mushrooms are very poisonous. Berries on wild plants are pretty, but many such berries are dangerous.

Know the names of the plants in and around your home. Do not have dangerous plants in children's play areas.

CALL THE POISON CENTER

If you think your child has swallowed or breathed something potentially poisonous, call the National Capital Poison Center immediately. You can reach the closest center at 800-222-1222.

FAMILY ACTIVITY

Assist your child in determining whether the items in the column below are food or not food, and place a check mark in the correct column to the right.

	EAT/DRINK	DON'T EAT/DRINK

What Drugs Can Do

LEARNING OBJECTIVES

- Children will communicate ways tobacco and alcohol are used.
- Children will state that smoking or chewing tobacco can affect our bodies.
- Children will state how alcohol can affect our bodies.

The intent of the activities in this chapter is to help children gain an awareness of tobacco and alcohol products and to provide a foundation for future decision making. Children learn healthy and unhealthy habits from observing and imitating adults and other children, both at home and at school. For example, when children observe adults smoking and drinking alcohol, they are likely to identify these substances and may view their use as typical adult behavior in social situations. Avoid making statements such as "smoking is bad," or "drinking is not smart." Such statements criticize many parents, adults, and family members and often confuse children. It is likely that many family members and other adults important to children do use tobacco and alcohol products; judging the behavior or the person is not appropriate.

The purpose of the activities in this chapter is to begin a discussion of the health and safety issues related to these products. Address alcohol and tobacco separately to avoid confusing children. To begin a discussion on tobacco, you may choose to show a tobacco plant and tell how it is grown. In some regions, some young children, as well as their family members, may be involved in growing this crop. Next, explain how the plant is used to make cigarettes, cigars, snuff, and chewing tobacco. When discussing the impact of tobacco (and alcohol) on the body, remember that children most relate to and understand what they can see and experience around them. For example, allowing children to hold a tobacco leaf or particles of tobacco from a cigarette helps them see that the tobacco does not produce negative effects through a single touch.

Use questions to encourage discussion, and allow children to share their experiences with people who use tobacco around them. Questions might include "How did it smell?" and "How did it look?" and "Was there smoke?" and "How did the smoke make you feel?" and "Was anything left when the person finished smoking the cigarette or the pipe?"

Often children will recognize the effect of smoke on their eyes (for example, their eyes burn or sting) and their sense of smell. Though children may have difficulty understanding how tobacco can cause harm to the lungs or heart since they cannot see the heart or lungs, discuss these effects and follow with activities that help children understand more clearly.

When introducing the topic of alcohol, first explain that it is a liquid that comes in various forms and is found in many products; then begin to identify products that contain alcohol. Examples include beverages such as beer, wine, and liquor. Help children understand that drinking alcohol is not always bad, but that too much alcohol inside the body can be harmful. Help children understand that drinking even small amounts of alcohol can be very dangerous for children. Children may have questions about other "alcohol" they have seen, such as the isopropyl alcohol used in first aid. Explain that these are different types of alcohol and they should never taste or drink these products.

Remember, children cannot control adult behavior or their home environment. Since alcohol and tobacco may be commonly used in families, show care and understanding when dealing with these topics. As children become more aware of the impact that various chemicals and products have on their bodies, they may become frightened for themselves or family members. Help parents and family members recognize the risk of these products to children. Secondhand smoke is especially harmful to young children and can lead to lower respiratory tract infection and fluid in the middle ear (for example, ear infections), and can aggravate symptoms in children with asthma, allergies, and other respiratory issues. Thirdhand smoke is the contamination that remains after the cigarette, cigar, or pipe has been put out. Smoke residue and odor remain on a smoker's skin, hair, and clothing; they also remain on furniture, carpets, and curtains for several days. These residual toxins can be harmful, especially to young children. Therefore, tobacco use of any type (for example, smoking) should not be allowed in areas to which children have access or where the fumes and toxins can enter children's areas (for example, through ventilation systems).

Children should not have access to a smoker's matches and lighters, for access can result in fire injury and death. Children also should not have access to alcohol products; even a single drink can cause life-threatening injury to a young child.

VOCABULARY

adult drink	container	label	secondhand smoke
advertisement	crop	mixed drink	smoking
alcohol	curing	nicotine	tobacco
beer	dipping	pesticide	warning
chewing tobacco	food preparation	pipe	wine
cigar	fuel	rubbing alcohol	
cigarette	irritated eyes		

CREATING THE ENVIRONMENT

- Prohibit smoking in all areas of the facility, including classrooms, offices, hallways, entrance areas, and outdoor play areas. A smoke-free facility reduces the impact of secondhand smoke on children.

- Prohibit smoking in vehicles that transport children.

- Make sure all field trips are to smoke-free areas.

- Remind family members and volunteers that smoking is not permitted in the program facility or children's areas (for example, on the playground). If a smoking area is needed for staff, provide it outdoors in an area where adults are completely out of children's view and where smoke cannot drift into children's areas. Check local and funding regulations regarding smoke-free environments.

- Keep playgrounds and entrances clear of debris, including alcohol or tobacco products and containers.

- Store any product containing alcohol in a locked cabinet.

EVALUATION

- Do children show awareness that smoking or chewing tobacco can affect our bodies (for example, smoke irritates eyes and causes coughing)?

- Do children show awareness that drinking alcohol can affect our bodies?

- In guided activities, can children recognize products containing tobacco?

- In guided activities, can children distinguish containers used for alcohol?

- In role play, do children reflect an understanding of the ways that tobacco and alcohol are used?

CHILDREN'S ACTIVITIES

The Tobacco Plant

Show children a tobacco plant (*Nicotiana*) and encourage them to look at it closely, touch it gently (because it is a living plant), and smell it. Ask if they know what it is. Tell them that it is called a tobacco plant, and ask what they have heard about tobacco. Listen to any comments they make, and consider them for future activities. Let children know that some farmers grow tobacco for their job and they sell it to people to use in many ways. Briefly explain that tobacco plants may be grown in yards like flowers, used in some medicines, and made into products for smoking and chewing.

MATERIALS
- a live tobacco plant

OTHER IDEAS

- Visit a tobacco farm, Skype with a tobacco farmer, or watch a video clip of a tobacco farm to see tobacco plants growing. Have the farmer demonstrate how to care for or process the plants at that stage. See if children can be engaged in the activity in any way. Ask the farmer to explain how the plants were started, what was done to care for the plants, and what will be done later. Arrange for children to see any equipment used in growing tobacco.

  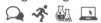

- Show children cigarettes, cigars, and chewing tobacco. In front of the children, break the paper on the cigarettes and cigars to show what is inside, and open the containers of chewing tobacco. Encourage children to feel and smell the products and to compare each of them. Talk about how feeling and smelling the tobacco a single time will not harm them.

- Provide tobacco plant seeds, and engage children in planting, caring for, and monitoring the growth of the plants.

- Arrange for children to see, feel, and smell cured tobacco, and compare the leaves to the growing plant leaves. Show pictures of the curing process, or invite a farmer to explain it to the children, including the time frame.

Tobacco Labels and Ads

Show children a cigarette, a cigar, chewing tobacco, and a pipe, and ask what each is. If children do not know, tell them and explain that each one uses tobacco. Let children see empty recreational tobacco containers, such as cigarette packages and cartons and chewing tobacco containers. Point out the variety of brands and kinds of containers. Ask children to cut out tobacco advertisements or any pictures of tobacco from magazines, catalogs, and newspapers you provide. Encourage children to show and talk about what they collected. Read aloud to children the labels from any ads they found and the containers you provided, including the warnings. Briefly explain that cigarettes contain a substance called nicotine and that it is addictive, which means that once a person begins smoking it is very hard to quit. Answer any questions they have simply, honestly, and in a nonjudgmental way.

MATERIALS

- cigarettes, pipes, cigars, chewing tobacco, tobacco product cartons and containers, magazines, catalogs, newspapers, and scissors

OTHER IDEAS

- Assist children in matching the advertisements and photographs they found to the containers provided for this activity. Point out that there are many brands and different looks for tobacco.

- Help children make a mosaic using one of their tobacco advertisements or pictures. Instruct them to cut the picture into about one-inch squares, one at a time. Show them how to glue each of the squares onto a piece of construction paper to make the picture whole again.

- Invite someone who has stopped smoking to visit and explain to the children why she stopped smoking and how hard it was. Ask the visitor to be honest but to focus on the positive reasons (like being able to breathe better and live longer) and to avoid frightening the children about loved ones dying because of smoking.

- Display a "no smoking" sign, and ask children where they might see one. Go for a walk in the program facility, and look for any no smoking signs.

Discuss briefly why smoking is not allowed at the program, and include that the end of a cigarette is a tiny fire that could burn children if they were to run into it.

Smoke Smells

Acquire clothes recently worn by a person who smokes or who was in a smoky environment. Place the clothes in a small suitcase or other container and close it tightly. Place freshly laundered clothes in another small suitcase or other container and close it tightly too. Show the children the two containers, and tell them they are going to participate in a smelling game, in which they will smell clothes from each suitcase and compare the odors. Gather children closely when each suitcase is opened, and invite them to sniff and describe what they smell. Let them know that one set of clothes was worn by a person who was near smoke, and ask if they can guess which one. Explain that smoke smells can stick to clothes, hair, and the body. Tell them that the smoke smell can come from cigarettes, pipes, cigars, bonfires, house fires, and cars or rooms where there is a smoke smell. Ask children to share about any time they have been where there was a strong smoke smell. Listen and reinforce any statements about smoke burning their eyes, making it hard to see, causing breathing to be difficult, making their nose stuffy, causing food to taste bad, or leaving a lingering smell. Explain that washing their face, opening a window, or covering their nose with their shirt sometimes helps.

MATERIALS

■ smoky-smelling clothes, fresh-smelling clothes, and two small suitcases

OTHER IDEAS

■ Invite someone to the classroom who is actively trying to stop smoking. Ask him to briefly tell the children why he wants to stop, to explain what he is doing to stop, and to describe how his body feels while he is trying to quit. Ask the guest if the smell of smoke was one of the reasons.

■ Visit a health clinic, health department, or doctor's office to have a health care professional briefly explain what happens to the smoke when someone smokes a cigarette. Ask the health professional to describe the effects the smoke has on the body, using charts, props, or displays appropriate for young children.

■ Play, sing, and dance to "No Tobacco" by Tickle Tune Typhoon in collaboration with the Comprehensive Health Education Foundation. Explain that children should not smoke or chew tobacco and that the song is for helping them remember that.

■ Provide supplies, and encourage children to make a picture of what smoke looks like. Remind children that smoke can come from many sources and that it is important to avoid breathing the smoke into their bodies when they can.

Shayla's Scrape

Show children a bottle of rubbing alcohol, and let them look at the container, see the alcohol being poured from the original container into a clear bowl, and smell the alcohol. Ask if they know what it is. Tell them that it is called rubbing alcohol, and ask what they have heard about it and other types of alcohol. Listen to any comments they make, and consider them for future activities. Let children know that rubbing alcohol can be used in many ways, but it is often used as a medicine to help clean cuts and scrapes. Let each child use a cotton ball dipped very lightly into the alcohol to clean an imaginary scrape on Shayla, a classroom doll, before tossing the ball into the trash. Tell children rubbing alcohol can be used to clean lots of things, like thermometers, mirrors, sticky stuff, and more. Briefly explain that there are many kinds of alcohol and that some kinds are used in various types of medicine, food preparation, fuel, and adult drinks (wine, beer, mixed drinks).

MATERIALS

■ rubbing alcohol container with alcohol, clear bowl, one cotton ball per child, and a classroom doll

OTHER IDEAS

■ Invite a health professional to talk about how rubbing alcohol is used in her job. Explain to children that rubbing alcohol is different from the alcohol used in adult beverages.

■ Invite a professional housekeeper who uses rubbing alcohol for cleaning to demonstrate cleaning a variety of items. Ask the housekeeper to explain to the children why he uses alcohol for cleaning.

■ Invite a chef who uses alcohol in food preparation to talk with children about why and how she uses alcohol when cooking. Explain that the alcohol burns off and does not affect our bodies. Ask the chef to use a measuring cup or spoon to show children the amount of alcohol used when cooking a meal.

■ Show a remote-control car. Explain to children that play cars and real cars have to run on some kind of energy. Tell them that some kinds of vehicles use a type of alcohol to make them go. Let children learn to operate the remote-control car.

Alcohol Labels and Ads

Show children empty, clean alcohol product containers. Point out the many brands, shapes of containers, and kinds of alcohol. Remind children about the ways various types of alcohol are sometimes used in medicine, food preparation, fuel, and adult drinks (wine, beer, mixed drinks). Ask children to cut out alcohol advertisements or any pictures or photographs of alcohol products from magazines, catalogs, and newspapers you provide. Encourage children to show and talk about what they collected. Read aloud to children the labels from any ads they found and the containers you provided, including any warnings. Answer any questions they have simply, honestly, and in a nonjudgmental way.

MATERIALS

- alcohol product containers (rubbing alcohol, mouthwash, cough syrup, cleansing products, and beverages), magazines, catalogs, newspapers, and scissors

OTHER IDEAS

- Assist children in matching the advertisements and pictures they found to the containers provided for the above activity. Point out that there are many brands and different looks for alcohol.

- Help children make a mosaic using one of their alcohol advertisements or pictures. Instruct them to cut the picture into about one-inch squares, one at a time. Show them how to glue each of the squares onto a piece of construction paper to make the picture whole again.

- Invite someone who has stopped drinking to visit and explain to the children why he stopped drinking and how hard it was. Ask the person to be honest but to focus on the positive reasons and to avoid frightening the children about loved ones who drink.

- Display a "No drinking alcohol allowed" sign or a warning sign about consuming alcohol. Place similar signs throughout the classroom, and encourage children to find them. Examples of warnings may be from beverage containers, hot tub and spa manuals, equipment, or medicine. Read to the children the signs they find and discuss them briefly.

Screen Time

Watch a carefully selected public service announcement about drinking at too young an age or about drinking and driving. Discuss the content with the children. Explain that some adult drinks contain alcohol and those drinks can be very dangerous for children, even big kids. Tell them that when adults drink too much, it can cause them to have bad breath, have trouble seeing and hearing, cause their body to move slower, make them sad, make them too loud, or make them say things they do not really mean. However, adults also can do all of those things and not have been drinking.

MATERIALS

- recording of public service announcement about underage drinking or about drinking and driving, and a viewing device for the video

OTHER IDEAS

- Invite a social drinker, who uses in moderation, to share with children why she does not drink too many alcoholic drinks at one time. Remind children that even when they drink too much water too fast, it can make their stomach ache. Help them understand terms like *a little* and *too much*.

- Invite someone to the classroom who is actively trying to stop drinking. Ask him to briefly tell the children why he wants to stop, to explain what he is doing to stop, and to describe how his body feels while he is trying to quit. Remind the person that the children are young and may misunderstand personal details or graphic examples.

- Visit a health clinic, health department, or doctor's office to have a health care professional briefly explain what happens to the alcohol when someone drinks it. Ask the health professional to describe the short-term effects alcohol has on the body (positive and negative) by using charts, props, or displays appropriate for young children.

- Assist children in making a video showing what they know about alcohol. If the video does not include private family information and it is appropriate, use it in parent training or send it to a local television or radio station to use as a public service announcement.

FAMILY INFORMATION

WHAT ALCOHOL CAN DO

The alcohol in beer, wine, cough syrup, mouthwash, and other products can be very dangerous for young children. Alcohol lowers the body's blood sugar and can cause illness, coma, or even death for a young child. Just a few sips of an alcohol product can cause serious problems for children.

Keep all alcohol products out of children's reach. If alcoholic beverages are served, empty all glasses and containers when finished. Do not leave alcoholic beverages where children may find them.

SECONDHAND SMOKE

Secondhand smoke is smoke from someone else's cigarette. It has harmful effects on everyone, especially children. Breathing smoke can lead to asthma, sinus and ear infections, allergies, and respiratory problems.

Teach your child that smoking hurts the body. If you smoke, avoid smoking in your car, home, or other closed places when children are present. Encourage other people to avoid smoking in front of your child. It may be hard to stop smoking. Encourage your child never to start smoking.

HEALTHY DECISIONS

Healthy habits and decision-making skills begin in early childhood. Begin teaching your child now to recognize tobacco and alcohol products. Your child should learn how to respond to invitations to smoke a cigarette, chew tobacco, or drink alcohol. Explain to your child the appropriate responses to such invitations.